普通高等教育"十一五"国家级规划教材
全国高等医药院校药学类实验双语教材

生药学实验与指导

（供药学类和中药学类专业用）

主　编　毕志明
副主编　刘惠娟
主　审　李　萍
编　委　（以姓氏笔画为序）
王冲之　王　铎　刘惠娟　毕志明
张体灯　李会军　贺清辉　顾晓洁
楚　楚　蒯玉花

U0786496

中国医药科技出版社

内 容 提 要

《生药学实验与指导》是全国高等医药院校药学类实验双语教材之一，与《生药学》课程的课堂教学配套使用。本书根据全国高等医药院校本科《生药学》教学大纲编写，以大纲规定的实验内容为主，并做了必要的补充与扩展，旨在使学生通过实验课的学习，能够灵活掌握生药学的基本概念、基本理论和实验的基本技能。同时增加了一些综合实验及实践，有意加强学生的独立动手能力、实验设计能力、综合实验能力及研究创新能力，从而提高学生独立思考和解决问题的良好素质。

本书可作为全国高等医药院校本、专科药学类和中药学类专业实验教学用书，也可作为有关专业的继续教育教材或自学教材的参考书。

图书在版编目（CIP）数据

生药学实验与指导：英汉对照/毕志明主编. —北京：中国医药科技出版社，2007. 2

全国高等医药院校药学类实验双语教材. 普通高等教育“十一五”国家级规划教材

ISBN 978 -7 -5067 -3602 -2

Ⅰ. 生…　Ⅱ. 毕…　Ⅲ. 生药学 - 实验 - 双语教学 - 医学院校 - 教材 - 英、汉　Ⅳ. R93 -33

中国版本图书馆 CIP 数据核字（2007）第 019676 号

美术编辑　陈君杞
责任校对　张学军
版式设计　郭小平

出版　中国医药科技出版社
地址　北京市海淀区文慧园北路甲 22 号
邮编　100082
电话　发行：010 - 62227427　邮购：010 - 62236938
网址　www. cmstp. com
规格　787 × 1092mm $^{1}/_{16}$
印张　12 $^{1}/_{2}$
字数　288 千字
版次　2007 年 2 月第 1 版
印次　2020 年 8 月第 7 次印刷
印刷　三河市国英印务有限公司
经销　全国各地新华书店
书号　ISBN 978 -7 -5067 -3602 -2
定价　20.00 元

出版说明

全国高等医药院校药学类专业规划教材是目前国内体系最完整、专业覆盖最全面、作者队伍最权威的药学类教材。随着我国药学教育事业的快速发展，药学及相关专业办学规模和水平的不断扩大和提高，课程设置的不断更新，对药学类教材的质量提出了更高的要求。

全国高等医药院校药学类规划教材编写委员会在调查和总结上轮药学类规划教材质量和使用情况的基础上，经过审议和规划，组织中国药科大学、沈阳药科大学、广东药学院、北京大学药学院、复旦大学药学院、四川大学华西药学院、北京中医药大学、西安交通大学医学院、华中科技大学同济药学院、山东大学药学院、山西医科大学药学院、第二军医大学药学院、山东中医药大学、上海中医药大学和江西中医学院等数十所院校的教师共同进行药学类第三轮规划教材的编写修订工作。

药学类第三轮规划教材的编写修订，坚持紧扣药学类专业本科教育培养目标，参考执业药师资格准入标准，强调药学特色鲜明，体现现代医药科技水平，进一步提高教材水平和质量。同时，针对学生自学、复习、考试等需要，紧扣主干教材内容，新编了相应的学习指导与习题集等配套教材。

本套教材由中国医药科技出版社出版，供全国高等医药院校药学类及相关专业使用。其中包括理论课教材 82 种，实验课教材 38 种，配套教材 10 种，其中有 45 种入选普通高等教育“十一五”国家级规划教材。

全国高等医药院校药学类规划教材
编写委员会
2009 年 8 月 1 日

序

实验教学是高等药学院校最基本的教学形式之一，对培养学生科学的思维与方法、创新意识与能力，全面推进素质教育有着重要的作用。飞速发展的科学技术，已成为主导社会进步的重要因素。高等药学院校必须不断更新教学内容，以学科发展的前沿知识充实实验课程内容。

近年来，中国药科大学坚持以研究促教改，通过承担教育部“世行贷款——21世纪初高等教育教学改革项目”及立项校内教改课题等多种方式，调动了广大教师投身教学改革的积极性，将转变教师的教育思想观念与教学内容、教学方法的改革紧密结合起来，取得了实效。此次推出的国家“十一五”规划教材——药学专业双语实验教学系列，是广大教师长期钻研实验课程教学体系，改革教学内容，实现教育创新的重要成果。他们站在21世纪教育、科技和社会发展趋势的高度，对药学专业实验课程的教学内容进行了“精选”、“整合”和“创新”，强调对学生的动手能力、创新思维、科学素养等综合素质的全面培养。这套教材具有以下的特点：

1. 教材将各学科的实验内容进行了广泛的“精选”，既体现了高等药学教育“面向世界、面向未来、面向现代化”，也考虑到我国药学教育的现状与实际；既体现了各门实验课程自身的独立性、系统性和科学性，又充分考虑到各门实验课程之间的联系与衔接，有助于学生在教学大纲规定的实验教学学时内掌握基本操作技术，提高动手能力，养成严谨、求实、创新的科学态度。

2. 教材中新增的综合性、设计性实验有利于学生全面了解和综合掌握本门实验课程的教学内容。这一举措既满足了学生个性发展的需要，更注重培养学生分析问题、解决问题的能力和创新意识。

3. 教材中适当安排一些反映药学学科发展前沿的实验，有利于学生在掌握实验基本技术的同时，对药学学科的新进展、新技术有所了解，激发他们学习药学知识与相关学科的兴趣。

4. 教材以实践教学为突破口，采用双语体系编写，为实验课程改革构建数字化、信息化和外语教学的平台，有利于提高学生的科技英语水平。通过我校多年的药学系列实验课程双语教学实践，证明学生完全能够接受此套教材的教学。

国家十一五规划教材——药学专业双语实验教学系列教材的陆续出版，必将对推动我国高等药学教育的健康发展，产生积极而深远的影响。由于采用双语体系编写药学教学实验丛书尚属首次，缺乏经验，在内容选择及编写方法上的不妥之处，在所难免。欢迎从事药学教育的同行们批评赐教。

吴晓明

（中国药科大学校长、博士、教授、博士生导师）

Preface

Experimental teaching is one of the most fundamental teaching means in pharmaceutical colleges, playing an important role in training scientific thoughts and methods, creative consciousness and ability of the students as well as in promoting quality-oriented education in all-round way. Fast-advancing science and technology has come to be an important factor in dominating social progress. Teaching materials must be updated continually in pharmaceutical colleges, especially enriching the materials of experimental courses with the most advanced knowledge in the subject.

In recent years, China Pharmaceutical University have been stressing the promotion of teaching reform on the basis of research, succeeding in stimulating teachers' enthusiasm for teaching reform by various means such as undertaking the project of teaching reform in higher education at the beginning of 21st century sponsored financially by World Bank and entrusted by the Ministry of Education as well as approving and ratifying internal programs on teaching reform. Meanwhile, it yields fruits to integrate the transforming of teachers' educational ideology into the reform of teaching materials and methods. This series of textbook of national "11th five" planning-bilingual pharmaceutical experimental teaching series, is an important achievement made through studying ueaching system of experimental courses for long, reforming teaching materials and carrying out educational innovation of all the teachers concerned.

Meeting the new demands for education, science and technology and social growth, they select, integrate and innovate the teaching materials of pharmaceutical experimental courses, stressing the overall cultivation of comprehensive qualities, including experimental ability, creative thought and scientific attainments. This set of textbook possesses the following features:

1. These textbooks make an extensive "selection" of the experimental materials of each subject, reflecting the goal of facing the world, facing the future and facing the modernization in higher pharmaceutical education, and taking into account the status quota and reality of our pharmaceutical education; meanwhile embodying the individuality, systematicness and scientificalness of each experimental courses, which helps the students to grasp basic techniques of operation within the class hours of experimental teaching pre-

scribed by teaching syllabus and to improve their experimental ability and finally to cultivate a scientific approach of precision, practicality and creation.

2. The comprehensive designing experiments newly supplemented in the textbooks help the students to learn totally and grasp comprehensively the teaching materials of the experimental courses, which not only meets the students' needs for individual development but also trains their ability to analyze and solve problems and cultivates their creative consciousness.

3. Some experiments representing the latest development in pharmacy are properly included in the textbooks, which helps the students to learn about new advance and technology in pharmacy and to further arouse their interests in studying pharmacy and relevant subjects while grasping some basic techniques of experiment.

4. The textbooks take experimental teaching as starting point and are compiled in a system of bilingualism and aim to set up a platform of digitalization, information and foreign language teaching for the purpose of reforming experimental courses, which serves to enhance the students' level of technological English. It has been proved that the students have no difficulty being adapted to the teaching of this set of textbook through many years of bilingual teaching practice carried out in a series of pharmaceutical experimental courses of our university.

The successive publishing of the series of textbooks used for bilingual pharmaceutical experimental teaching-the national "11th-five" planning textbooks, will surely produce good and far-reaching influence in promoting the sound development of higher pharmaceutical education of our country. Since it is the first time that we have compiled this series of textbook of pharmaceutical teaching experiment in a bilingual system, we lack experience and thus some defects in choice of materials and way of compilation are inevitable. Experts engaged in pharmaceutical education are welcome to give any criticisms and advice.

Wu Xiaoming

Ph. D, prof., and supervisor of doctoral candidates
President of China Pharmaceutical University

前　言

《生药学实验与指导》是全国高等医药院校药学类实验双语教材之一，与《生药学》课程的课堂教学配套使用。本书根据全国高等医药院校本科《生药学》教学大纲编写，以大纲规定的实验内容为主，并做了必要的补充与扩展，旨在使学生通过实验课的学习，能够灵活掌握生药学的基本概念、基本理论和实验的基本技能。同时增加了一些综合实验及实践，有意加强学生的独立动手能力、实验设计能力、综合实验能力及研究创新能力，从而提高学生独立思考和解决问题的良好素质。

本书分为总论和各论两大部分。总论部分主要为生药的理化分析、生药中水分及灰分的测定、生药中挥发油及浸出物的含量测定等。各论部分主要为代表性科属生药的实验内容，包括生药的性状、显微鉴别、理化鉴别、含量测定等内容。全书共编有36个实验，使用时可根据各自的教学安排逐个进行或灵活删并。每个实验后的实验作业，也可根据各自的需要给以改动。

本教材为中、英文双语教材，每一实验的中文部分在前，英文部分在后，文中的插图均编排在中文部分。

本教材的编写得到了中国医药科技出版社、中国药科大学的大力支持和资助；楚楚、易玲、夏黎、王伟、钱正明、李沁等研究生协助主编做文字校对等工作，在此一并致以深深的谢意。

本书为全国医药院校本科、专科的实验教学用书，也可作为有关专业的继续教育教材或自学教材的参考书。

由于时间和水平所限，教材中存在的缺点和错误在所难免，恳切希望应用本教材的广大师生和读者批评指正。

编　者

2006年12月于中国药科大学

Preface

Experiment and Guide for Pharmacognosy is one of the bilingual experimental teaching material and to be used together with the classroom teaching textbook *Pharmacognosy*. This textbook is compiled on the basis of syllabus of *Pharmacognosy*. In order to let the students master the basic concept, theory and skills better, some necessary supplements were added. Synthetic experiments and practice were also compiled in the book on the purpose of enhancing the comprehensive ability of the students, such as independent practice, experiment design, creative research, and hopefully to result in the students' good diathesis of independent thinking and solving problems.

This book is divided into two sections. Physical and chemical identification, contents determination of water, ash, essential oil and extracts, etc, are included in the general notes. The specified experiment of each crude drug in representative family includes its description, microscopic, physical and chemical identification, contents determination, etc. There are totally 36 experiments in this textbook, and the experiments and assignments could be arranged orderly or freely since necessary.

As a bilingual textbook, Chinese of each experiment is laid out completely with the illustrations before the English text.

Without the labor and financial supports from Chinese Medical and Technology Press and China Pharmaceutical University, this book couldn't be achieved its publication. In addition, post - graduates as Chu Chu, Yi Ling, Xia Li, Wang Wei, Qian Zhengming, Li Qin, etc helped the editor a lot during the compilation. We would like to show our sincere acknowledgments to them.

This textbook is mainly used in experimental teaching for specialized students and undergraduates in medical universities, and yet also suitable for continuing education and self-taught study.

Limited by time and level, there must be mistakes in the book. So criticism and constructive suggestions are welcome.

Editors

China Pharmaceutical University

Dec. 2006

目　　录

Contents

实验一　生药的理化分析（一）

【实验目的】

1. 掌握生药中糖类、苷类化学成分的理化性质和定性反应，并能应用于生药鉴定中，以确证生药中这些成分是否存在。

2. 了解糖类及苷类主要鉴别反应的反应原理。

【实验材料】

党参 Radix Codonopsis、苦杏仁 Semen Armeniacae Amarum、槐花 Flos Sophorae、大黄 Radix et Rhizoma Rhei、夹竹桃叶 Folium Thevetiae、桔梗 Radix Platycodi、牡丹皮 Cortex Moutan、白芷 Radix Angelicae Dahuricae、柴胡 Radix Bupleuri。

【实验方法】

1. 单糖、多糖与苷类成分的鉴别

取党参 0.5 g，剪碎，置 50 ml 三角烧瓶中，加蒸馏水 10 ml，瓶口放一小漏斗（空气冷凝，防止水分蒸发太多），水浴温热数分钟，滤过，药渣中加适量水，再滤过，合并滤液至 10 ml，备用。

（1）费林试验（Fehling 试验）：取滤液 1 ml 于 50 ml 烧杯中，加碱性酒石酸铜试剂（Fehling 试剂）8 ml（临用时由甲液与乙液等量混合而成，置沸水浴加热 5 分钟，观察有无砖红色沉淀产生（如有沉淀，表明含还原糖），在整个反应过程中，反应液应保持蓝色，否则应适当添加 Fehling 试剂至蓝色不褪，继续加热 5 分钟，放冷，滤过，滤液加 10% 盐酸，使反应液的 pH 为 1～2，再在沸水浴加热 10 分钟（水解），放冷，加 10% 氢氧化钠试液，使反应液呈中性，再加 Fehling 试剂 8 ml，沸水浴加热数分钟，观察有无砖红色沉淀产生（如有沉淀，表明含多糖或苷类）。记录水解前后沉淀量的多少（以“+ + +”示很多，“+ +”示较多，“±”示很少来表示）。

（2）α－萘酚试验（Molisch 试验）：取滤液 1 ml 于大试管中，加 α－萘酚试剂 2～3 滴，摇匀，沿管壁缓缓滴加浓硫酸 1 ml，轻放试管架上，保留两层液面，观察两液面交界处有无形成紫红色环。

2. 氰苷的鉴别

（1）苦味酸钠试验：取苦杏仁粗粉约 0.5 g，置具塞试管中，加水适量湿润，管内悬挂一条苦味酸钠试纸，密塞，将试管置 60℃ 水浴中温热，观察试纸逐步由黄色变为砖红色。

（2）普鲁士蓝试验：取苦杏仁粗粉约 0.5 g 置试管中，加水少许湿润，立即用滤纸包扎管口，滤纸用 1～2 滴氢氧化钾试液湿润，将试管置 60℃ 水浴温热约 10 分钟后，于试纸上加硫酸亚铁溶液 1 滴，并加稀盐酸和 5% 三氯化铁试液各 1 滴，滤纸即显蓝色。

3. 酚苷的鉴别

取牡丹皮粗粉 0.5 g，加乙醇 5 ml，水浴温热 5 分钟，取上清液 2 ml 于试管中，滴加 1%三氯化铁试剂 1 滴，即呈紫红色。

4. 蒽苷的鉴别

（1）Bontrager 反应：取大黄粉 0.1 g 于小试管中，加 10%氢氧化钠试液 2 ml，振摇，溶液即呈红色，滤过，滤液加 10%盐酸使中和，溶液变黄色；加入乙醚 2 ml，振摇使之分层，醚液呈黄色，吸取醚液层置另一试管中，加氢氧化钠试液 1 ml，振摇后碱液又显红色。

（2）醋酸镁反应：取大黄粉末约 0.2 g 于试管中，加乙醇 3 ml，水浴温热 5 分钟，滤过，得滤液，加 1%醋酸镁甲醇溶液 2 滴，振摇后观察，溶液渐呈橙红色。

（3）微量升华：如图 1－1 所示，取大黄粉末少许于金属圈内，小火徐徐加热数分钟，可见黄色升华物附着载玻片上，将玻片取下翻转后，在显微镜下检视，低温升华时可见针状结晶、高温时可见羽毛结晶，滴加碱液后，结晶消失，并呈红色。

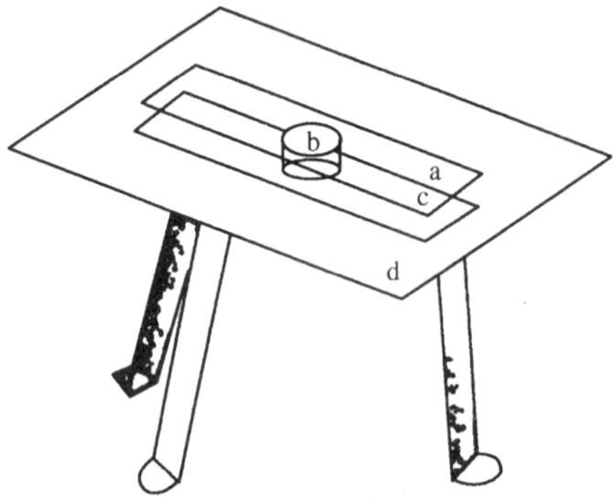

图 1－1 微量升华装置

a. 载玻片 b. 金属圈 c. 金属片 d. 中有小孔的石棉板

5. 黄酮苷类的鉴别

取槐米粗粉 0.5 g，加乙醇 10 ml，水浴温热 5 分钟，滤过，得滤液。

（1）盐酸－镁粉还原反应：取上述滤液 2 ml 于试管中，先滴加浓盐酸 2～3 滴，再加镁粉少许振摇，产生许多气泡，同时溶液渐变樱红色。

（2）三氯化铝反应：取上述滤液 2 ml 于试管中，加 1%三氯化铝甲醇溶液 1 ml，振摇，可见溶液渐变鲜黄色。

6. 皂苷的鉴别

取桔梗粗粉 1 g，置 50 ml 三角烧瓶中，加生理盐水 15 ml，在水浴上加热 20 分钟，滤过。滤液作以下（1）、（2）试验。

（1）泡沫试验：取上述滤液 2 ml，置试管中，密塞或以手指压住管口，强烈振摇数分钟，观察是否产生大量泡沫，放置 10 分钟后，再记录泡沫的高度。

（2）溶血试验：将 2%红细胞悬浮液滴于载玻片上，盖上盖玻片，置显微镜下，观察红细胞形状，然后于盖玻片边缘滴加桔梗滤液，观察有无溶血现象。如红细胞破裂溶解，为阳性反应。

（3）Libermann 反应：取柴胡粗粉 1 g，置锥形瓶中，加 70%乙醇 10 ml，于水浴中温热数分钟，滤过，滤液置蒸发皿中，水浴蒸干，放冷，加醋酐 1 ml 使溶解，并转入小试管中，沿管壁加浓硫酸 1 ml，两液面的交界处显紫红色环。

7. 强心苷的鉴别

取夹竹桃叶粗粉 2 g，加 70%乙醇 15 ml，再加 10%醋酸铅 2 ml，在水浴上煮沸 5 分钟，滤过，得滤液，作下列试验。

（1）Keller－Kiliani 反应：取夹竹桃滤液 2 ml 于蒸发皿中，水浴蒸干，加三氯化铁－冰醋酸试液 1 ml 使残渣溶解，并转入小试管中，沿管壁缓缓滴加浓硫酸 1 ml，观察两液层交界处有无棕色环产生，冰醋酸层显蓝绿色（α－去氧糖反应）。

（2）Kedde's 反应：取滤液 5ml，加新配制的3,5－二硝基苯甲酸乙醇溶液 1 ml，溶液显紫红色（强心苷苷元上的五元不饱和内酯环的反应）。

8. 香豆精苷的鉴别

异羟肟酸铁反应：取白芷粗粉 0.5 g，置具塞试管中，加乙醚 3 ml，振摇 5 分钟后，静置约 20 分钟，取上清液 1 ml 于另一试管中，加 7%盐酸羟胺甲醇溶液与 20%氢氧化钾甲醇溶液各 2～3 滴，摇匀，置水浴上微热，冷却后，加稀盐酸调节 pH 至 3～4，再加 1%三氯化铁乙醇溶液 1～2 滴，溶液呈紫红色。

【实验作业】

记录各鉴别反应的步骤与结果，并说明反应原理（可用化学反应式表示）。

【思考题】

1. Fehling 反应中，水解前后产生 Cu_2O 沉淀的主要成分是什么？
2. 怎样鉴别某生药含单糖、多糖或苷类中的糖成分？
3. 具有什么基团的蒽醌类成分与氢氧化钠溶液反应才显红色？为什么？
4. 如何区别某生药所含皂苷是三萜皂苷还是甾体皂苷？
5. 异羟肟酸铁反应开始时，加碱性试剂的作用是什么？

1 Physico-chemical Identification of Crude Drugs (Ⅰ)

Objectives

1. Master the physico-chemical properties and qualitative reactions of carbohydrates and glycosides in crude drugs, and ascertain these constituents in the crude drug identification.

2. Study the principle of the main identification reactions of carbohydrates and glycosides.

Experiment Material

Radix Codonopsis, Semen Armeniacae Amarum, Flos Sophorae, Radix et Rhizoma Rhei, Folium Thevetiae, Radix Platycodi, Cortex Moutan, Radix Angelicae Dahuricae, Radix Bupleuri.

Experiment Methods

1. Identification of monosaccharides, polysaccharides and glycosides

Cut Radix Codonopsis into fragments to a 50 ml conical flask, add 10 ml of distilled water, put a little funnel on the flask (avoid water's evaporation), warm in water bath for several minutes, filter, add some water to gruffs, filter again, combine filter liquor to 10 ml for preparation.

(1) Fehling's Test: add 1 ml of filter liquor and 8 ml Fehling agent in a 50 ml beaker, warm on a boiled water bath for 5 minutes, observe whether a brick-red precipitate is produced (if the precipitate is produced, contained reductive sugar), during the whole reaction, blue colour was maintained, otherwise add Fehling agent until blue colour is unchanged, continue to heat for 5 minutes, chill, filter, add 10% hydrochloric acid until pH is 1 to 2, continue to warm on a boiled water bath for 10 minutes (hydrolysis), chill, add 10% NaOH test solution to pH = 7, then add 8ml Fehling agent, continue to warm on a boiled water bath for several minutes, observe whether a brick-red precipitate is produced. Record the quantity precipitation of before and after the hydrolysis. ("+ + +" show much; "+ +" show some; "±" show little)

(2) Molisch's Test: add 1 ml of filter liquor and 2 or 3 drops of α－naphthol to a

big tube, shake well-distributed, slowly add 1ml of concentrated sulphuric acid along tubal wall, put it on tube-carrier gently, maintain two layers of liquor, observe in two liquors' b oundary whether a violet-red verge is produced.

2. Identification of cyanogenic glycosides

(1) Sodium picrate test: add 0.5 g of amygdala amara's coarse powder to a test tube with a cork, moisten with several drops of water, hang a strip of sodium picrate test paper, stopper tightly, put the tube on a 60℃ water bath, observe test paper changing colour from yellow to brick-red gradually.

(2) Prussian blue test: add 0.5 g of amygdala amara's coarse powder to a tube, moisten with several drops of water, and bandage canal orifice right now, to 1 or 2 drops of KOH test solution moisten filter paper, put the tube on a 60℃ water bath for 10 minutes, add a drop of ferrous sulfate test solution, 5% chloride ferric and dilute hydrochloric acid respectively, then filter paper shows blue colour.

3. Identification of phenol glycosides

Add 5 ml of ethanol to 0.5 g of Cortex Moutan's coarse powder, warm on water bath for 5 minutes, to 2 ml supernatant to tube, add a drop of 1% chloride ferric, a violet-red colour is produced.

4. Identification of anthra glycosides

(1) Bontrager test: add 0.1 g of rhubarb's coarse powder and 2 ml of 10% NaOH test solution to a tube, shake well-distributed, test solution shows red, filter, add 10% hydrochloric acid to counteract, yellow colour is produced; add ether, shake into delamination, the ether layer shows yellow, imbibe the ether layer to another tube, add 1 ml NaOH TS, after joggle, the lye layer shows red again.

(2) Magnesium acetate test: add 0.2 g of rhubarb's coarse powder and 3 ml of ethanol to a tube, warm on water bath for 5 minutes, filter, add 2 drops of 1% magnesium acetate test solution to filtrate, shake, a orange-red colour is produced.

(3) Microamount sublimation: add a little rhubarb's coarse powder into metal ring, heat it with tiny flame for several minutes, yellow sublimate. Accrete on microscope slide, take microscope slide under microscope, needle crystal can be seen at low temperature, and feather crystal can be seen at high temperature, add lye to them, crystal disappear, a red colour is produced.

5. Identification of flavonoid glycosides

Add 10ml ethanol to 0.5 g of Flos Sophorae's coarse powder, warm on water bath for 5 minutes, filter, get the filtrate.

(1) Hydrochloric acid-magnesium reductive test: add 2ml above-mentioned filtrate to a tube, firstly add 2 or 3 drops of concentrated hydrochloric acid into it, then put some magnesium to reduce decompose, shake, many bubbles produce, and a herry-red

colour is produced.

(2) Aluminum trichloride test: add 2 ml above-mentioned filter to a tube, add 1ml of 1% Aluminum trichloride in methanol, shake, a daffodil colour is produced.

6. Identification of saponins

Add 1 g of Radix Platycodi's coarse powder and 15 ml of normal saline to a 50 ml conical flask, warm on water bath for 20 minutes, filter.

(1) Foam test: add 2 ml of above-mentioned filter to a tube, close canal orifice tightly with stopper, or press it with finger, shake it strongly for several minutes, observe whether a lot of loam is produced, stand for 10 minutes, then record the height.

(2) Haematolysis test: carry 2% erythrocyte soliquoid on microscope slide under microscope, observe the shape of erythrocyte, then drop Radix Platycodi's filter liquor to the edge of microscope slide, observe whether the phenomenon of haematolysis is produced. If erythrocyte resolved, test is positive reaction.

(3) Libermann test: Add 1 g of Radix Bupleuri's coarse powder and 10 ml of 70% ethanol to a conical flask, warm on water bath for several minutes, filter. put the filtrate into evaporating basin, warm on water bath to dry, chill, add 1ml of acetic anhydride to dissolve, transfer it to a small tube, add some concentrated sulphuric acid along tube wall, observe two liquors' boundary whether a violet-red verge is produced.

7. Identification of cardiac glycosides

To 2 g of Folium Thevetiae's coarse powder, add 15 ml of 70% ethanol and 2 ml of 10% lead acetate solution, warm on a boiled water bath for 5 minutes, filter.

(1) Keller-Kiliani test: put 2 ml of filtrate into an evaporating basin, warm on water bath to dry, add 1ml of chloride ferric in glacial acetic acid to dissolve, transfer it to a small tube, add some concentrated sulphuric acid along tube wall, observe two liquors' boundary whether a brown verge is produced, glacial acetic acid layer shows blue-green colour.

(2) Kedde's test: to 5 ml of above-mentioned filtrate, add 1 ml of neo-prepared 3,5-dinitro-benzoic acid in ethanol, a voilet-red colour is produced.

8. Identification of coumarins

Ferric hydroxamic test: add 0.5 g of Radix Angelicae Dahuricae's coarse powder and 3 ml of ether to a tube with a cork, shake for 5 minutes, stand about 20 minutes. To 1 ml clear supernatant add 2 or 3 drops of 7% hydroxylamine hydrochloride in methanol and 20% carstic potash in methanol respectively in another tube, shake to uniformity, warm on a water bath, chill, add hydrochloric acid to adjust pH to 3 or 4, then add 1 or 2 drops of 1% chloride ferric in ethanol in ethanol, a violet-red colour is produced.

Laboratory Assignments

Record the procedure and result of each identification, and state the principle (demonstrated by chemical equation).

Questions

1. In Fehling test, what're the main constituents for cuprous oxide precipitation before and after the hydrolysis?

2. How to identify monosaccharides, polysaccharides and glycosides in some crude drugs?

3. What's the reason about appearance of red colour when caustic soda solution meets anthraquinone with some certain groups, and what're the groups?

4. How to distinguish the saponins in some crude drugs whether triterpenoid saponins or steroidal saponins?

5. At the beginning of the reaction of ferric hydroxamic test, what's the purpose of adding alkalinity agent?

实验二　生药的理化分析（二）

【实验目的】

1. 掌握生药中生物碱、鞣质、氨基酸和蛋白质的理化性质和定性反应，并能应用于生药鉴定中，以确证生药中这些成分是否存在。

2. 了解主要鉴别反应的反应原理。

【实验材料】

百部 Radix Stemonae、马钱子 Semen Strychni、五倍子 Galla Chinensis、儿茶 Catechu、天花粉 Radix Trichosanthis。

【实验方法】

1. 生物碱的鉴别

取百部粗粉 1 g，置 50 ml 三角烧瓶中，加 1%盐酸 15 ml、振摇 15 分钟，滤过。将滤液分装于 6 支小试管中，每试管 1 ml，其中一支作为空白对照，其余分别滴加下表中生物碱沉淀剂各 2 滴，观察沉淀的颜色与数量（以 + + +、+ +、+ 表示）。

沉淀剂 样品	碘化铋钾	碘－碘化钾	碘化汞钾	硅钨酸	鞣酸
百部提取液	橘红色沉淀	棕色沉淀	白色沉淀	灰白色沉淀	浅棕黄色沉淀

2. 鞣质类的鉴别

分别取五倍子与儿茶粗粉 2 g，加水 20 ml，40～50℃水浴加热 20 分钟，冷却，滤过，五倍子滤液和儿茶滤液分别各置 5 支试管，依次加入下述试剂，观察溶液变化。

试剂	五倍子（可水解鞣质）	儿茶（缩合鞣质）
醋酸铅试液	乳白色沉淀	淡黄色沉淀，易溶于稀醋酸
新配制的饱和石灰水	青灰色沉淀	棕色或红棕色沉淀
饱和溴水	无沉淀	黄色或橙红色沉淀
三氯化铁试液	溶液显蓝色或蓝黑色并有沉淀	溶液显绿色或绿黑色或沉淀

3. 氨基酸与蛋白质的鉴别

取天花粉粗粉 0.5 g，加 50%乙醇 10 ml，水浴加热 10 分钟，滤过，得滤液并加水至 10 ml，备用。

（1）茚三酮反应（Niuhydrin 反应）：取滤液 1 ml 于试管中，加新配制的茚三酮试剂 2 滴，水浴加热数分钟，观察颜色反应。另取小滤纸，滴加滤液 1 滴，吹干，再滴加茚三酮试剂 1 滴，用电吹风烘烤，观察颜色变化。

（2）双缩脲反应（Biuret 反应）：取滤液 4 ml 于试管中，加 10% 氢氧化钠试液 2 滴，继加 0.5% 硫酸铜试液 2 滴，振摇并静置，观察溶液颜色变化。溶液显蓝色为阳性反应。

【实验作业】

记录各鉴别反应的步骤与结果，并说明反应原理（可用化学反应式表示）。

【思考题】

1. 如何确证某一生药中存在生物碱类成分？
2. 写出可水解鞣质与缩合鞣质的鉴别反应。
3. 如何鉴别生药中存在的是氨基酸还是蛋白质？

2 Physico-chemical Identification of Crude Drugs (Ⅱ)

Objectives

1. Master the physico-chemical properties and qualitative reactions of alkaloids, tannins, amino acid and proteins in crude drugs, and identify the drugs through examining the existence of these constituents.

2. Study the principles of the main identification reactions.

Experiment Material

Radix Stemonae, Semen Strychni, Galla Chinensis, Catechu, Radix Trichosanthis.

Experiment Methods

1. Identification of alkaloids

Add 1 g of coarse-powdered Radix Stemonae and 15 ml of 1% hydrochloric acid solution into Erlenmeyer flask. Shake for 15 minutes and filter. Transfer filtrate into 6 test tubes respectively, 1 ml in each one, and take one of them as the blank test. To the rest add 2 drops of alkaloid-precipitants respectively as the following table shows. Observe the color and quantity of the precipitate. (the quantity denoted with +++, ++, +)

Precipitant / Sample	potassium iodobismuthaste	potassium iodide-iodine	potassium mercuric iodide	silicotungstic acid	Tannins
extract of Radix Stemonae	orange-red precipitate	brown precipitate	white precipitate	off-white precipitate	light brown-yellow precipitate

2. Identification of tannins

To 2 g of coarse-powdered of Galla Chinensis and Catechu add 20 ml of water respectively. Warm on a water bath at 40～45℃ for 20 minutes, allow to cool and filter. Transfer the filtrate of Galla Chinensis and Catechu to 5 test tubes respectively, add the following reagents consequently. Observe the changes of the solutions.

Reagents	Galla Chinensis (hydrolysable tannins)	Catechu (condensed tannins)
Plumbic acetate TS	Cream white precipitate, undissolved in dilute acetic acid	Light yellow precipitate, dissolved in dilute acetic acid
Fresh saturated calcareous water	Green-gray precipitate	Brown or reddish-brown precipitate
Saturated bromic water	No precipitate	Yellow or orange-red precipitate
Ferric chloride TS	Solution shows blue or blue-black and produces precipitate	Solution shows green or green-black or produces precipitate

3. Identification of amino acids and proteins

To 0.5 g of coarse-powdered Radix Trichosanthis add 10 ml of 50% ethanol. Warm on a water bath for 10 minutes and filter. To the filtrate add water to 10 ml, ready for using.

(1) Ninhydrin Reaction: Place 1 ml of filtrate in a test tube, add 2 drops of fresh Ninhydrin reagent, warm on a water bath for several minutes, and observe the color reaction. Apply 1 drop of the drug solution to a piece of small filter paper, blow to dry, then apply 1 drop of Ninhydrin reagent, blow with drier. Observe the changes of color.

(2) Biuret Reaction: Place 4 ml of the drug solution in a test tube, apply 2 drops of 10% NaOH TS firstly, then add 2 drops of 0.5% vitriolum veneris TS, shake and stand. Observe the color changes of the solution. That the solution produces blue is a positive reaction.

Laboratory Assignments

Record the procedure and result of each identification reaction and indicate the principles of reactions (demonstrated by chemical equations).

Questions

1. How to confirm the existence of alkaloids in crude drugs?
2. State the identification reactions of hydrolysable tannins and condensed tannins.
3. How to identify the existence of amino acids or proteins in crude drugs?

实验三　生药中水分及灰分的测定

【实验目的】

1. 掌握烘干法及甲苯法测定生药中水分含量的方法，了解减压干燥法测定水分含量的方法。

2. 掌握生药中总灰分与酸不溶性灰分的测定方法。

3. 了解生药中水分、总灰分与酸不溶性灰分测定的意义。

【实验材料】

大青叶 Folium Isatidis、当归 Radix Angelicae Sinensis、大黄 Radix et Rhizoma Rhei。

【实验方法】

1. 烘干法测定水分

取大青叶碎片(直径不超过 3 mm)约 5 g,平铺于干燥至恒重的扁形称重瓶中,厚度不超过 10 mm,精密称定重量(W_1),打开瓶盖在 100～105℃ 干燥 5 小时,将瓶盖盖好,移置干燥器中,冷却 30 分钟,精密称定重量,再在上述温度干燥 1 小时,冷却,称重,至连续两次称重的差异不超过 5 mg 为止(W_2)。根据减失的重量,计算样品中含有水分的百分数。

$$生药中水分含量（\%）=\frac{W_1-W_2}{W_1}\times 100\%$$

2. 甲苯法测定水分

(1) 如右图安装仪器。

(2) 洗净全部仪器，置干燥箱内烘干，备用。

(3) 将甲苯置分液漏斗中，加少量水充分振摇，放置，分去水层，甲苯蒸馏后备用。

(4) 取当归粗粉适量（相当于含水量 2～4 ml），精密称定，置 A 瓶中，加甲苯约 200 ml，必要时加玻璃珠数粒，将仪器各部分按图连接，自冷凝管顶端加入甲苯，至充满 B 管的狭细部分。将 A 瓶置电热套中或用其他适宜方法缓缓加热，待甲苯开始沸腾时，调节温度，使每秒钟馏出 2 滴。待水分完全馏出，即测定管刻度部分的水量不再增加时，将冷凝管内部分先用适量甲苯冲洗，再用饱蘸甲苯的长刷或其他适宜的方法，将管壁上附着的甲苯推下，继续蒸馏 5 分钟，放冷至室温，拆卸装置，如有水黏附在 B 管上，可用蘸甲苯的铜丝推下，放置，使水分与甲苯完全分离。读取水量，并换算成样品中含有水分的百分数（V/W）。

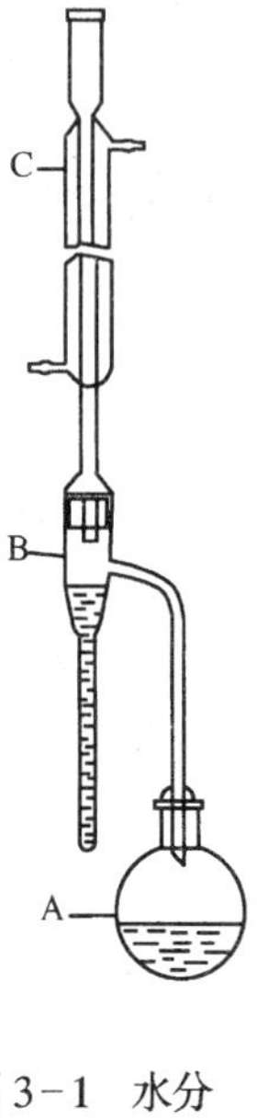

图 3-1　水分测定器(甲苯法)

A. 圆底烧瓶

B. 水分测定管

C. 直形冷凝管

$$生药中水分含量（\%）=\frac{水量（ml）}{样品重量（g）}\times 100\%$$

3. 总灰分的测定

取大黄粗粉 3～5 g（如不需测定酸不溶性灰分，可取供试品 2～3 g），置已炽灼至恒重的坩埚中，称定重量（准确至 0.01 g），缓缓炽灼，注意避免燃烧，至完全炭化时，逐渐升高温度至 500～600℃，使完全灰化并至恒重。根据残渣重量，计算大黄中含灰分的百分数。

$$生药中总灰分含量（\%）=\frac{残渣重量}{供试品重量}\times 100\%$$

4. 酸不溶性灰分的测定

取上项所得的灰分，在坩埚中小心加入稀盐酸 9～11 ml，用表面皿覆盖坩埚，置水浴上加热 10 分钟，表面皿用热水 5 ml 冲洗，洗液并入坩埚中，用无灰滤纸滤过，坩埚内的残渣用水洗于滤纸上，并洗涤至洗液不显氯化物反应为止。滤渣连同滤纸移至同一坩埚中，干燥，炽灼至恒重。根据残渣重量，计算供试品中含酸不溶性灰分的百分数。

$$生药中酸不溶性灰分含量（\%）=\frac{酸处理并烧灼后残渣重量}{供试品重量}\times 100\%$$

【实验作业】

1. 分别记录大青叶与当归的水分测定过程，并计算它的水分含量。
2. 记录灰分测定实验步骤，并分别计算大黄中总灰分与酸不溶性灰分的含量。

【思考题】

1. 试述甲苯法测定生药中水分的原理。
2. 试述测定酸不溶性灰分的意义与原理。

3 Determination of Water and Ash in Crude Drugs

Objectives

1. Master two methods, drying in oven method and toluene distillation method, and study the drying under reduced pressure method, to determine the content of water in crude drugs.

2. Master the methods to determine the content of total ash and acid-insoluble ash in crude drugs.

3. Study the significance of determining the content of water, total ash and acid-insoluble ash in crude drugs.

Experiment Material

Folium Isatidis, Radix Angelicae Sinensis, Radix et Rhizoma Rhei.

Experiment Methods

1. Drying in oven method to determine the content of water

Place 5 g of pieces of Folium Isatidis (with less than 3 mm in diameter) being examined in a flat weighing bottle, previously dried to constant weight, to form a smooth layer not exceeding 10 mm in thickness and then accurately weigh (W_1). Dry in an oven at 100 ~ 105℃ for 5 hours with the stopper of the bottle removed. Upon opening the oven, close the bottle promptly and allow it to cool in a desiccators for 30 minutes. Weigh accurately and dry it again under similar condition for 1 hour, cool and weigh. Repeat the operation until the difference between two successive weights is not more than 5 mg (W_2). Calculate the percentage content of water in the substance being examined according to the weight loss on drying.

$$\text{The content of water in crude drugs (\%)} = \frac{W_1 - W_2}{W_1} \times 100\%$$

2. Toluene distillation method to determine the content of water

Place a quantity of the powered Radix et Rhizoma Rhei being examined which is anticipated to yield about 2 ~ 4 ml of water and accurately weighed, in the flask A. Add about 200 ml of toluene and a few glass beads if necessary. Assemble the apparatus as the picture shows and fill the receiving tube B with toluene through the top of condenser until the graduated portion is full. Heat the flask gently. When toluene begins to boil, adjust the temperature and allow to distill at a rate of 2 drops per second. When the volume of water in the receiving tube does not increase any more, rinse the inside of condenser with toluene and push down the toluene adhering to the wall with a brush or other suitable tools. Continue the distillation for 5 minutes. Cool to room temperature and disconnect the apparatus. Push down any droplet of water adhering to the wall of the receiving tube with a copper wire wetted with toluene. Allow to stand until water is completely separated from toluene in the receiving tube. Record the volume of water distilled and calculate the percentage of water in the substance being examined.

$$\text{The content of water in crude drugs (\%)} = \frac{\text{the volume of water (ml)}}{\text{the weight of sample (g)}} \times 100\%$$

3. Determination of total ash

Place 3~5 g (2~3 g if not for the determination of acid-insoluble ash) of powered Radix et Rhizoma Rhei in a tared crucible. Weigh accurately (to nearest 0.01 g), ignite slowly till the sample is completely carbonized. Keep it from burning with care. raise the temperature gradually to 500~600 ℃. Incinerate to constant weight and the ash is carbon-free. Calculate the percentage of ash with reference to the air-dried drug.

$$\text{The content of water in crude drugs (\%)} = \frac{\text{the weight of air-died drug}}{\text{the weight of sample}} \times 100\%$$

4. Determination of acid-insoluble ash

Place the ash obtained in the determination of total ash in a crucible, add 9~11 ml of dilute hydrochloric acid with great care, cover with a watch glass. Heat on a water bath for 10 minutes. Rinse the watch glass with 5 ml of hot water and add the rinsings to the crucible. Filter with an ashless filter paper, transfer the residue to the filter paper with water, wash till the filtrate yields no reactions of chlorides. Transfer the filter paper together with the residue to the original crucible, dry and ignite to constant weight. Calculate the percentage of acid-insoluble ash with reference to the air-dried drug.

$$\text{The content of acid-insoluble ash in crude drugs(\%)} = \frac{\text{the weight of residue dealt by acid and then ignite}}{\text{the weight of sample}} \times 100\%$$

Laboratory Assignments

1. Record the procedure of the water determination in Folium Isatidis and Radix Angelicae Sinensis respectively, and calculate the content of water in them.

2. Record the procedure of ash determination, calculate the content of total ash and acid-insoluble ash in Radix et Rhizoma Rhei respectively.

Questions

1. Try to state the principle of the toluene distillation method in determining the content of water in crude drugs.

2. Try to state the meaning and principle of determining the acid-insoluble ash.

实验四 生药中挥发油及浸出物的含量测定

【实验目的】

1. 掌握生药中挥发油含量测定的方法。
2. 掌握常用的测定生药中浸出物含量的方法。
3. 了解生药中挥发油、浸出物含量测定的意义。

【实验材料】

薄荷 Herba Menthae、巴戟天 Radix Morindae Officinalis、续断 Radix Dipsaci、连翘 Fructus Forsythiae、杜仲 Cortex Eucommiae、独活 Radix Angelicae Pubescentis。

【实验方法】

1. 挥发油的测定

根据挥发油的相对密度大小不同，挥发油的测定有甲、乙两种方法。甲法适用于测定相对密度在1.0以下的挥发油，乙法适用于相对密度在1.0以上的挥发油。

(1) 甲法

取薄荷（约5 mm的碎段）适量（约相当于含挥发油0.5～1.0 ml），称定重量（准确至0.01 g），置烧瓶中，每100 g供试品加水600 ml与玻璃珠数粒，振摇混合后，连接挥发油测定器与回流冷凝管。自冷凝管上端加水使充满挥发油测定器的刻度部分，并溢流入烧瓶时为止，置电热套中或其他适宜的方法缓缓加热至沸，并保持微沸约3小时，至测定器中油量不再增加，停止加热，放置片刻，开启测定器下端的活塞，将水缓缓放出，至油层上端到达刻度0线上面约5 mm处为止。放置1小时以上，再开启活塞使油层下降至上端恰与刻度0线平齐，读取挥发油体积，并计算样品中含挥发油的百分数（V/W）。

$$样品中挥发油的含量（\%）=\frac{测得的挥发油体积（ml）}{样品重量（g）}\times 100\%$$

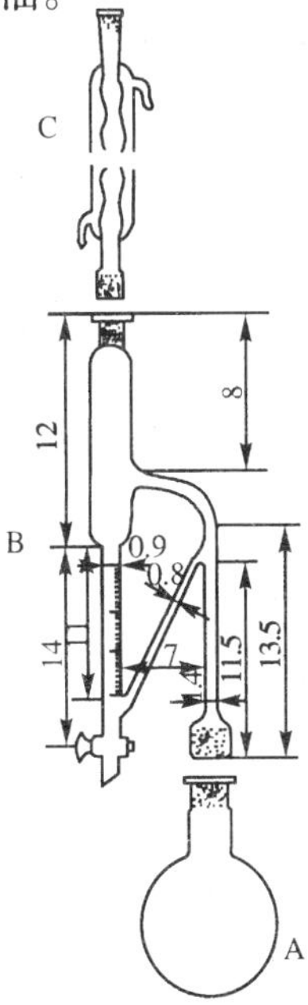

图4-1 挥发油测定装置(长度单位为cm)

A. 圆底烧瓶

B. 挥发油测定器

C. 球形冷凝管

(2) 乙法

取水约300 ml与玻璃珠数粒，置烧瓶中，连接挥发油测定器。自测定器上端加水充满刻度部分，并溢流入烧瓶时为止，再用移液管加入二甲苯1 ml，然后连接回流冷凝管。将烧瓶内容物加热至沸腾，并继续蒸馏，其速度以保持冷凝管的中部呈冷却状态为度。30分钟后，停止加热，放置15分钟以上，读取二甲苯的体积。然后照甲法自“取供试品适量”，依法测定，自油层体积中减去二甲苯的体积，即为挥发油体积，再计算供试品中含挥发油的百分数。

$$样品中挥发油的百分含量（ml/g）=\frac{油层体积(ml)-二甲苯体积(ml)}{样品重量（g）}\times 100\%$$

2. 浸出物的测定

对于有效成分尚不明确或尚无精确定量方法的生药，一般可根据已知成分的溶解性能，选用适宜的溶剂，提取并测定生药中可溶性浸出物的含量，用以表示该生药的质量。

常用的溶剂有水、一定浓度的乙醇和乙醚 3 种。通常采用冷浸法和热浸法进行测定。

供测定的生药样品粉末除另有规定外，应能通过二号筛，并混合均匀。

（1）水溶性浸出物的测定

①冷浸法：取巴戟天粗粉约 4 g，称定重量（W，准确至 0.01 g），置 250 ml 锥形瓶中，精密加入蒸馏水 100 ml，密塞冷浸，前 6 小时内时时振摇，再静置 18 小时，用干燥滤器迅速滤过，精密吸取滤液 20 ml，置于已干燥至恒重的蒸发皿中，在水浴上蒸干，于 105℃ 干燥 3 小时，移置干燥器中，冷却 30 分钟，迅速精密称定重量（W_1），按干燥品计算生药中含水溶性浸出物的百分数。

$$生药中水溶性浸出物含量（\%）=\frac{W_1\times 100}{20\times W}\times 100\%$$

②热浸法：同上法取续断粉末 4 g 于 250 ml 锥形瓶中，精密加入蒸馏水 100 ml，塞紧，称定重量（W，准确至 0.01 g），静置 1 小时后，连接冷凝管，加热至沸腾，并保持微沸 1 小时，放冷后，取下锥形瓶，密塞，称定重量，用水补足减失的重量，摇匀，用干燥滤器滤过。精密吸取滤液 25 ml，置已干燥至恒重的蒸发皿中，在水浴上蒸干，于 105℃ 干燥 3 小时，移置干燥器中，冷却 30 分钟，迅速精密称重，按干燥品计算生药中含水溶性浸出物的百分数。

（2）醇溶性浸出物的测定

醇溶性浸出物的测定亦有冷浸法和热浸法两种，其测定方法与水溶性浸出物的测定法相同，只是用不同浓度的乙醇或甲醇代替水为溶媒。乙醇或甲醇的浓度，《中国药典》在各被测品种项下均有规定。热浸法需在水浴上加热。

①冷浸法：取连翘粉末约 4 g，称定重量（准确至 0.01 g），照水溶性浸出物的冷浸法测定，以 65% 乙醇代替水。

②热浸法：取杜仲粉末约 4 g，称定重量（准确至 0.01 g），照水溶性浸出物的热浸法测定，以 75% 乙醇代替水（需在水浴上加热）。

（3）醚溶性浸出物的测定

取独活粉末约 2 g（通过四号筛），在五氧化二磷干燥器中放置 48 小时，称定重量（准确至 0.01 g），置 100 ml 索氏提取器中，加乙醚 70 ml，水浴加热回流提取 4 小时，放冷，过滤，以少量乙醚冲洗烧瓶及回流器，洗液与滤液合并至 100 ml 容量瓶中，加乙醚至刻度，摇匀。精密量取 50 ml 置已干燥至恒重的蒸发皿中，水浴低温蒸去乙醚，移至五氧化二磷干燥器中放置 24 小时，取出，迅速精密称重，计算样品中含醚溶性浸出物的含量。

【实验作业】

简要记录所测生药中挥发油和浸出物的测定步骤，并计算含量。

【思考题】

1. 测定挥发油的过程中，影响测定结果的因素有哪些?
2. 什么样的生药需测定浸出物含量?

4 Determination of Volatile Oil and Extractives

Objectives

1. Master the method of determining the content of volatile oil in crude drugs.

2. Master the method usually used for determining the content of extractives in crude drugs.

3. Study the significance of determining the content of volatile oil and extractives in crude drugs.

Experiment Material

Herba Menthae, Radix Morindae Officinalis, Radix Dispsaci, Fructus Forsythiae, Cortex Eucommiae, Radix Angelicae Pubescentis.

Experiment Methods

1. Determination of volatile oil

Because of difference in the relative density, the determination of volatile oil has two methods. Method A is used for determining volatile oil of which the relative density is less than 1.0, and Method B is used for determining volatile oil of which the relative density is more than 1.0.

Method A Place proper quantity of Herb Menthae (5 mm segments in diameter), weigh accurately to the nearest 0.01 g (The weight of the drug being examined equivalent to 0.5～1.0 ml of volatile oil) into flask A. Add 600 ml of water per 100 g of the drug and a few glass beads, shake and mix well. Connect flask A to volatile oil determination tube B and then connect B to reflux condenser C. Add water through the top of reflux condenser C until the graduated tube of B is filled and water overflows to flask A. Heat the flask gently in an electric heating jacket or by other suitable means until boiling begins, continue heating for about 3 hours, until the volume of oil does not increase. Stop heating, allow to stand for a few minutes, and open the stopcock at the lower part of B, run off the water layer slowly until the oily layer is 5 mm above the zero mark. Allow to stand for at least 1 hour, open the stopcock again, run off the remaining water layer carefully until the oily layer is just on the zero mark. Read the volume of oil in the graduated portion of the tube and calculate the content of volatile oil, expressed as percentage (V/W).

$$\text{The content of volatile oil in the drug (\%)} = \frac{\text{the volume of volatile oil (ml)}}{\text{the weight of the drug (g)}} \times 100\%$$

Method B Transfer 300 ml of water and a few glass beads to flask A, connect flask A to volatile oil determination assembly B. Add water through the top of B until the graduated tube of B is filled and water overflows to flask A. Add 1 ml of xylene with a pipette and then connect the reflux condenser C to B. Heat the flask until boiling begins and continue the distillation at a rate that will keep the middle part of the condenser cold. Stop heating after 30 minutes, allow to stand for at least 15 minutes. Read the volume of xylene in the graduated portion of the tube, Carry out the procedure described under Method A, beginning at the words "Place proper quantity of...". Subtract the volume of xylene previously observed from the volume of the oily layer, the remainder is taken to be the content of volatile oil in the drug being examined, expressed as percentage.

$$\text{The content of volatile oil in the drug(ml/g)} = \frac{\text{the volume(the oily layer-xylene)(ml)}}{\text{the weight of the drug(g)}} \times 100\%$$

2. Determination of extractives

The crude drug whose effective ingredients is uncertain or can not be measured accurately and precisely, can be extracted with the proper solvent selected by the dissolvability of the known constituents in crude drug. Extracting and determining the soluble extractives can show the quality of the crude drug.

The solvents usually used contain water, ethanol and ether at certain concentration. Cold maceration method and hot maceration method are often used for determining.

Pulverize the material being examined pass through a NO. 2 sieve, unless other specified, mix well.

(1) Determination of water-soluble extractives

Cold maceration method Place 4 g of the powered Radix Morindae officinalis, weighed accurately (to the nearest 0.01 g) (W), in a 250 ml stoppered conical flask, add accurately 100 ml of water, and stopper well. Macerate the drug with shaking for 6 hours and allow to stand for 18 hours. Filter rapidly through a dry filter, transfer accurately 20 ml of filtrate to an evaporating dish, previously dried to constant weight, and evaporate to dryness on a water bath. Dry at 105℃ for 3 hours and allow to cool for 30 minutes in a desiccator. Weigh rapidly and accurately (W_1), calculate the percentage of water-soluble extractives with reference to the dried drug.

$$\text{The content of water-soluble extractives (\%)} = \frac{W_1 \times 100}{20 \times W} \times 100\%$$

Hot maceration method Place 4 g of the powered Radix Dispsaci weighed accurately (to the nearest 0.01 g) in a 250 ml stoppered conical flask, add accurately 100 ml of water, stopper well and weigh, allow to stand for 1 hour, connect flask to condense. Boil gently under reflux for 1 hour. Allow to cool, take off the flask, stopper well and weigh, add water to restore its original weight, shake well and filter through a dry filter. Place 25 ml of the filtrate, accurately measured, in an evaporating dish, previously dried to constant weight, and evaporate to dryness on a water bath. Dry at 105℃ for 3 hours and allow to cool for 30 minutes in a desiccator. Weigh rapidly and accurately, calculate the percentage of water-soluble extractives with reference to the dried drug.

(2) Determination of alcohol-soluble Extractives

The determination of alcohol-soluble extractives also includes hot maceration and cold maceration. The procedure is identical to that of the water-soluble extractive except that the different percentage of ethanol or methanol is used as solvent instead of water. The percentage of ethanol or methanol is specified under the drugs being examined in China Pharmacopoeia. Hot maceration should be heated on a water bath.

①Cold maceration method

To about 4 g of the powdered Fructus Forsythiae weighed accurately (to the nearest 0.01 g), carry out the determination of water-soluble extractives, cold maceration method, using 65% ethanol instead of water.

②Hot maceration method

To about 4 g of the powdered Cortex Eucommiae, weighed accurately (to the nearest 0.01 g), carry out the determination of water-soluble extractives, hot maceration method, using 75% ethanol instead of water. (Heated on a water bath)

3. Determination of ether-soluble extractives

Place about 2 g of powdered Radix Angelicae Pubescentis (through NO. 4 sieve), stored in phosphorus pentoxide desiccant for 48 hours, weighed accurately (nearest to 0.01 g). Place the powder in Soxhlet extractor. Add 70 ml of sulfuric ether heating on a water bath under reflux for 4 hours, cool and filter, rinse the flask and extractor with a little volume of ether, combine the washings and filtrate into a 100 ml volumetric flask, and dilute with ether to the volume, mix well. Place 50 ml of the filtrate, accurately measured, in an evaporating dish, previously dried to constant weight. Evaporate the ether extraction to dryness on a water bath at low temperature, transfer the residue to the desiccator containing phosphorus pentoxide, store for 24 hours, take out the residue, weigh rapidly and accurately, calculate the content of ether-soluble extractives in the sample

Laboratory Assignments

Record concisely the procedure of determining the volatile oil and extractives in the crude drugs being examined, and calculate the content.

Questions

1. During determining volatile oils, what are the elements that affect determining results?

2. What kinds of crude drugs need to be determined their quantity of extraction?

实验五　浙贝母总 DNA 的提取

【实验目的】

1. 了解 DNA 分子标记技术在生药鉴定中的应用。
2. 提取浙贝母新鲜叶中的总 DNA 用于 PCR 扩增等其他分子生物学实验。

【实验材料】

浙贝母 *Fritillaria thunbergii* Miq.。

【实验方法】

一、药品试剂

液氮；1×CTAB 缓冲液（含有 2%CTAB，1.4 mol/L NaCl，20 mmol/L EDTA，100 mmol/L Tris·HCl，pH 8.0）；三氯甲烷/异戊醇（24:1）或水饱和的苯酚/三氯甲烷（1:1）；RnaseA；异丙醇；70%乙醇；超纯水；TE 缓冲液：10 mmol/L Tris·HCl。

二、仪器设备

天平；研钵；微量移液枪（200～1000 μl，20～200 μl，1～20 μl）；移液枪枪头；1.5 ml Eppendorf 管；高速冷冻离心机；水浴锅。

三、操作步骤

1. 将新鲜浙贝母叶片在流水下冲洗，擦干。取 100 mg 材料，剪碎后放入研钵中，加入液氮快速研磨。

2. 将粉末转移入 1.5 ml Eppendorf 管中，迅速加入 65℃ 预热的 1×CTAB 缓冲液 1 ml，放入 65℃ 水浴中温育 15 分钟，并不时轻轻地颠倒离心管使混合均匀。

3. 在混合液中加入等体积的三氯甲烷/异戊醇（24:1）或苯酚/三氯甲烷（1:1），轻轻颠倒离心管几次使管内成乳浊液，4℃，8000r/min 离心 10 分钟使分层。

4. 将上清液转移至干净的离心管中，加入 1/100 体积的 RNaseA，颠倒混匀，37℃ 保温 30 分钟。

5. 加入 0.6 倍体积的异丙醇，仔细混匀，－20℃ 放置 1 小时沉淀 DNA。

6. 4℃，12 000r/min 离心 15 分钟，弃上清液，沉淀用 70% 乙醇洗 2 次，室温下挥干，加入 TE 缓冲液 50～100 μl 溶解。

7. 取 8 μl 反应产物进行琼脂糖凝胶电泳，然后在凝胶成像仪中观察扩增结果。

【实验作业】

记录实验步骤与结果。

【实验指导】

1. 原理

将植物材料在液氮中研磨使细胞内容物释放出，在去污剂如 CTAB 的作用下使 DNA 释放到提取缓冲液中，大部分蛋白质可通过苯酚或三氯甲烷抽提后变性、沉淀除去。上清液加入异丙醇沉淀收集 DNA。

2. 注意事项

（1）离心管、枪头、除酶以外的试剂都要经过灭菌，以防被 DNA 污染。

（2）用三氯甲烷/异戊醇（24∶1）或苯酚/三氯甲烷（1∶1）抽提蛋白质这一步操作可以重复几次，直至两液面间几无乳化层。

（3）DNA 沉淀物干燥时间不能过长，以免影响 DNA 的溶解。

5 Extraction of Total DNA of *Fritillaria thunbergii*

Objectives

1. Study the application of DNA molecular tag technology in crude drug's identification.

2. Extraction of *Fritillaria thunbergii* total DNA from fresh leaves and using the total DNA to other molecular experiments such as PCR etc.

Experiment Material

Fritillaria thunbergii Miq.

Experiment Methods

1. Reagent

Liquid nitrogen; 1×CTAB buffer (Containing 2% CTAB, 1.4 mol/L NaCl, 20 mmol/L EDTA, 100 mmol/L Tris·HCl, pH 8.0); Chloroform-isopentanol (24:1) or water-saturated phenol-chloroform (1 : 1); RNase A; Isopropanol; 70% ethanol, ultrapure water; TE buffer: 10mmol/L Tris·HCl.

2. Apparatus

Balance, Mortar, Micropipette (200~1000 μl, 20~200 μl, 1~20 μl), Pipette tips, Eppendorf tube (1.5 ml), High speed freeze centrifuge, Water bath.

3. Operating procedure

(1) Wash fresh leaves with flowing water, and wipe off water. Take 100 mg of material and cut into pieces. Grind materials in liquid nitrogen to powder promptly.

(2) Transfer powder into a 1.5 ml eppendorf tube and add 1ml of 1 × CTAB solution 65℃ heated before. The mixed solution was incubated for 15 min at 65℃ and reverse eppendorf tube gently from time to time in order to mix well.

(3) Add equal volume of chloroform-isopentanol (24:1) or phenol-chloroform (1:1), reverse gently several times and the blending become milky solution, 4℃, 8000r/min centrifuge for 10 minutes to separate.

(4) Transfer supernatant to a new tube, add 1/100 volume of RNase A, mix well and incubate for 30 minutes at 37℃.

(5) Add 0.6 volume of isopropanol and mix gently, then keep for 1h at −20℃.

(6) 4℃, 12 000r/min centrifuge for 15 minutes. Discard the supernatant wash the sediment with 70% ethanol for 2 times. Volatilize in room temperature and dissolve total DNA with 50～100 μl of TE solution.

(7) Load 8 μl of total DNA solution in a agarose gel. Electrophoretic separation was performed and the resulting DNA fragments were visualized by UV transillumination.

Laboratory Assignments

Record the procedure and result of this experiment.

Experiment Directions

1. Principle

Grind plant materials in liquid nitrogen, to release the content in the cell, with the use of decontaminant such as CTAB release DNA into TE buffer, and the majority of protein is discarded because of denaturation and precipitation after being extracted by phenol or chloroform. To supernatant add isopropanol to precipitate and collect DNA.

2. Items of Note

(1) The tube, tips and reagent except enzymes should be sterilized, to protect DNA from pollution.

(2) The process of extracting protein with chloroform-isopentanol (24∶1) or phenol-chloroform (1∶1), can be repeated for several times, until there is nearly no emulsion layer between two phases.

(3) The time for drying precipitation of DNA can't be too long, lest influence the dissolution of DNA.

实验六　浙贝母 r－DNA 的 ITS 区序列扩增

【实验目的】

1．了解 DNA 分子标记技术在生药鉴定中的应用。

2．扩增浙贝母的 r－DNA 的 ITS_1、5.8S、ITS_2 区的一段大约 700bp 的 DNA 片段。

【实验材料】

实验五中提取的浙贝母 DNA 产物。

【实验方法】

1．药品试剂

引物 P_1 和 P_2（各 10 pmol/μl）；10 mmol/L dNTPs；模板 DNA：约 0.05～1 μg 基因组 DNA；Taq DNA 聚合酶；10×PCR 缓冲液（500 mmol/L KCl，15 mmol/L $MgCl_2$，100 mmol/L Tris·HCl，pH 8.3）；超纯水；电泳所需试剂。

2．仪器设备

PCR 扩增仪；电泳装置；微量离心机；微量移液枪（20～200 μl、1～20 μl）；移液枪枪头；0.2 ml Eppendorf 管；凝胶成像仪。

3．操作步骤

（1）准备 PCR 反应溶液：

10×PCR 缓冲液	3 μl
dNTPs	0.6 μl
引物 P_1，P_2	各 1 μl
Taq DNA 聚合酶	1 U
模板 DNA	1 μl
超纯水	补足体积至 30 μl

（2）将反应管放入 PCR 仪中，按下列程序进行扩增反应：

①95℃预变性 5 分钟

②95℃ 30 秒

53℃ 40 秒

72℃ 60 秒

循环 30 次

③72℃延伸 10 分钟

反应结束后产物置 4℃保存。

（3）取 5 μl 反应产物进行琼脂糖凝胶电泳，然后在凝胶成像仪中观察扩增结果。

【实验作业】

记录实验步骤与结果。

【实验指导】

1. 原理

聚合酶链式反应（PCR）通常需要两个位于待扩增片段两侧的寡聚核苷酸引物，这些引物分别与待扩增片段的两条链互补，使两引物之间的区域得以通过聚合酶链式反应而扩增。扩增过程是：DNA 受热变性、引物与相应互补序列退火结合、接着在 DNA 聚合酶作用下进行延伸，如此重复多轮，由于延伸后得到的产物同样可与引物结合，因而每一轮循环后模板 DNA 的量都可加倍，于是位于两引物之间的 DNA 片段将以指数形式扩增。

2. 注意事项

（1）所有用具在实验前都要进行消毒以防止污染。

（2）设立对照组，以便出现问题时查找原因。

6 The Extension of r－DNA ITS Sequence of *Fritillaria thunbergii*

Objectives

1. Study the application of molecular tag technology in the area of crude drug's identification;

2. Extend about 700bp DNA fragments in ITS_1, 5.8S and ITS_2 areas of r－DNA of *Fritillaria thunbergii* Miq.

Experiment Material

DNA extractive of *Fritillaria thunbergii* Miq. in Experiment 5.

Experiment Methods

1. Reagent

Primer P_1 and P_2 (10 pmol/μl respectively); 10 mmol/L dNTPs; template DNA: about 0.05～1 μg of genomic DNA; Taq DNA polymerase; 10 × PCR buffer (500 mmol/L KCl, 15 mmol/L $MgCl_2$, 100 mmol/L Tris·HCl, pH 8.3); ultrapure water; reagents used in electrophoresis.

2. Apparatus

PCR amplification instrument, electrophoresis instrument, microcentrifuge, micropipette (20～200 μl, 1～20 μl), pipette tips, 0.2 ml Eppendorf tube, image maker of gel.

3. Procedure

(1) Prepare the PCR reaction solution

10 × PCR buffer	3 μl
dNTPs	0.6 μl
Primer P_1 and P_2	1 μl respectively
Taq DNA polymerase	1 U
template DNA	1 μl
ultrapure water	add the ultrapure water to 30 μl

(2) Put the reaction tube into the instrument of PCR, amplify according to the following procedure.

① Predenature at 95℃ for 5 min.

② 95℃ 30 s

53℃ 40 s

72℃ 60 s

Recycle 30 times.

③ Extending for 10 min at 72℃. The product stored at 4℃ after reaction.

(3) Load 5 μl of reaction product in a agarose gel, separation is performed and results of extension is visualized by the image maker of gel.

Laboratory Assignments

Record the experimental procedure and results.

Experiment Directions

1. Principle

Polymerase chain reaction (PCR) generally needs two oligonucleotide primers that flank the target region in duplex DNA. The primers are complementary to the fragments being extended. The primers are then extended on the template strand by using DNA polymerase. The extending procedure is that: denaturation of the DNA, achieved by heating the reaction, each primer binding with the complementary fragments after annealing, and the primers then extended by using a DNA polymerase. The cycle can repeat many times , the newly synthesized strand after extending can also bind with the primer, so that the amount of template DNA will double after every cycle, result in the exponential accumulation of a discrete fragment.

2. Items of note

(1) All apparatus should be sterilized in order to inhibit pollution before experiment.

(2) Set the control group in order to easily solve the problems in the experiment.

实验七　菌类生药——冬虫夏草的鉴定

【实验目的】

1. 掌握冬虫夏草性状及显微的主要鉴别特征。

2. 了解冬虫夏草类似品亚香棒虫草和凉山虫草与冬虫夏草在性状和显微特征上的主要区别点。

3. 了解冬虫夏草常见的伪品及其鉴别方法。

【实验材料】

冬虫夏草［冬虫夏草菌 *Cordyceps sinensis*（Berk.）Sacc. 寄生在蝙蝠蛾科昆虫幼虫上的子座及幼虫尸体的复合体］、亚香棒虫草 *C. hawkesii* Gary、凉山虫草 *C. liangshanensis* Zhang, Liu et Hu 的生药标本及样品。

【实验方法】

1. 性状鉴别

（1）冬虫夏草　由虫体和从虫头部长出的真菌子座相连而成。虫体似蚕，长3～5 cm，直径0.3～0.8 cm；头部红棕色，胸腹部深黄色或黄棕色，表面有20～30个环纹，腹面有足8对，以中部4对较明显；质脆，断面淡黄白色。子座1个，少数2～3个，细长圆柱形，稍扭曲，长4～7 cm，直径约0.3 cm；表面深棕色至棕褐色，有细纵皱纹，上部稍膨大，有不孕顶端；质柔韧，断面类白色，似纤维状。气微腥，味微苦。

（2）亚香棒虫草　虫体棕褐色，有40个环纹，腹足5对明显。子座1～2个，灰白色至灰褐色，无不孕顶端。

（3）凉山虫草　虫体棕褐色，直径6～10 mm，足不明显。子座有的上部分枝，长10～30 cm，直径1～2 mm，子囊壳突出于表面，有不孕顶端。

2. 显微鉴别

（1）冬虫夏草　取子座头部作横切面徒手切片：子囊壳近表面生，基部陷于子座内，椭圆形或卵圆形，直径140～245 μm，内有多数子囊。子囊细长，长240～485 μm，直径12～16 μm，顶部壁厚，中央有一狭线状孔口，子囊内有子囊孢子2～4个；孢子线形，长160～470 μm，直径约6 μm，有多数横隔。

（2）亚香棒虫草　同法作横切面徒手切片：子囊壳埋于子座内，长270～275 μm，直径94～192 μm。

（3）凉山虫草　同法作横切面徒手切片：子囊突出于子座外，长400～740 μm，直径27～40 μm，1～8个分泌细胞；柄1～3个细胞。

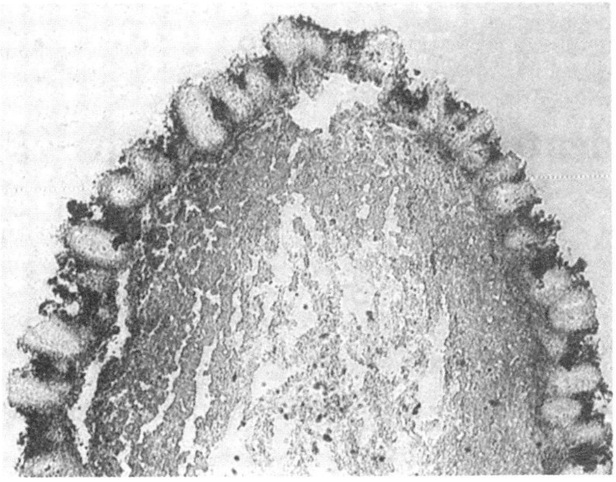

图 7－1　冬虫夏草横切面

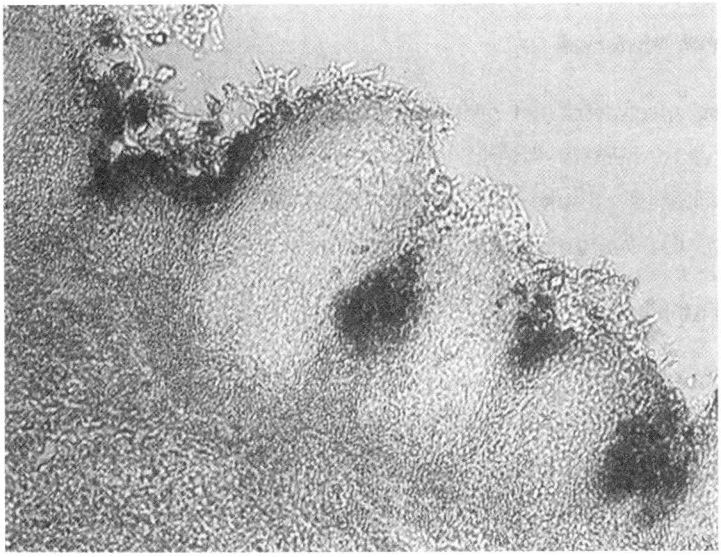

图 7－2　冬虫夏草横切面（局部放大）

【实验作业】

记述三种虫草的鉴别特征，列出三种虫草的显微特征检索表。

【思考题】

1. 曾有人以僵蚕、玉米粉或黄豆粉加染料模压制品伪充冬虫夏草，如何鉴别这些伪品？

2. 冬虫夏草的主要活性成分是什么？

3. 冬虫夏草在临床上有什么医疗价值？

7 Identification of Cordyceps (Fungi)

Objectives

1. Master the description and microscopic identification of Cordyceps.

2. Study main distinctions of description and microscopic identification between Cordyceps and *C. hawkesii* Gary, *C. liangshanensis* Zhang, Liu et Hu which analogous to Cordyceps.

3. Study usual adulterants of Cordyceps and their identification.

Experiment Material

Crude drug specimens of Cordyceps [a composite consisting of the stroma of the fungus, *Cordyceps sinensis* (Berk.) Sacc. (Fam. Hypocreaceae), parasitized on the larva of some species of insects (Fam. Hepialidae), and the dead caterpillar], *C. hawkesii* Gary, *C. liangshanensis* Zhang, Liu et Hu.

Experiment Methods

1. Description

(1) Cordyceps: a dead caterpillar jointed with a stroma growing in the head of the larva. The caterpillar resembling a silkworm, 3~5 cm long, 0.3~0.8 cm in diameter; head reddish-brown, the thorax and abdomen deep yellow or yellowish-brown, the surface with 20~30 annulations, on the abdomen feet 8 pairs, the 4 pairs in the middle relatively conspicuous; texture fragile, fracture pale yellowish-white. Stromata 1, minorities with 2~3 stromata, slenderly cylindrical, slightly twisted, 4~7 cm long, about 0.3 cm in diameter; externally deep brown to brown with fine longitudinal wrinkles, slightly swollen above, with infertility top, texture flexible; fracture whitish, fibrous-like. Odour , fleshy; taste, slightly bitter.

(2) *C. hawkesii*: caterpillar brown, with 40 annulations, feet on the abdomen 5 pairs conspicuous. 1~2 stromata, grayish-white to greyish-brown, without infertility top.

(3) *C. liangshanensis*: caterpillar brown, 6 ~ 10 mm in diameter, feet unconspicuous. Stromata sometimes branched above, 10~30 cm long, 1~2 mm in diameter, perithecium projecting out of surface, with infertility top.

2. Microscopic identification

(1) Cordyceps: transvers section of the head with a razor blade, perithecium grows near the surface, the base trapped in stroma, elliptical or oval, 140 ~ 245 μm in diameter, containing numerous ascus. Ascus slender, 240~485 μm long, 12~16 μm in diameter, walls thick in the top, in the center a narrow lined hollow, in ascus 2~4 spores; spores linear, 160~470 μm long, about 6 μm in diameter, with numerous trabeculas.

(2) *C. hawkesii*: transverse section as above with a razor blade, perithecium buried in stroma, 270~275 μm long, 94~192 μm in diameter,.

(3) *C. liangshanensis*: transverse section as above with a razor blade, ascus projecting out of stroma, 400~740 μm long, 27~40 μm in diameter. Secretory cells 1~8; stalk with 1~3 cells.

Laboratory Assignments

Record the identification of the three kinds of Cordyceps, list the microscopic identification of the three Cordyceps.

Questions

1. Using mechanograph of Bombyx batryticatus, corn powder or yellow bean powder and dyestuffs to simulate Cordyceps, how to identify these adulterants?
2. What are the main active principles of Cordyceps?
3. What are the clinical medical values of Cordyceps?

实验八　菌类生药——茯苓的鉴定

【实验目的】

1. 掌握茯苓的性状和显微的主要鉴别特征。
2. 掌握茯苓的理化鉴别方法。

【实验材料】

茯苓 *Poria cocos*（Schw.）Wolf 的生药标本（茯苓个、茯苓皮、茯苓块）及粉末。

【实验方法】

1. 性状鉴别

（1）茯苓个　呈类球形、椭圆形或不规则团块，大小不一。外皮薄，棕褐色或黑褐色，粗糙，具皱纹及缢缩，有时部分剥落。质坚实，破碎面颗粒性，近边缘淡红色，有细小蜂窝样孔洞，内部白色，少数粉红色，有的中间抱有松根。气微，味淡，嚼之粘牙。

（2）茯苓皮　呈不规则片状，外面棕褐色至黑褐色，内面白色或淡棕色，质较松软，略具弹性。

（3）茯苓块、茯苓片　多呈方形或长方形块片，白色、淡红色或淡棕色，平滑细腻。

2. 显微鉴别

茯苓粉末：①用斯氏液装片，可见无色不规则形颗粒团块、末端钝圆的分枝状团块及细长菌丝；遇水合氯醛液黏化成胶冻状，加热团块物溶化；②用 5% 氢氧化钾溶液装片，可见菌丝细长，稍弯曲，有分支，无色（内层菌丝）或带棕色（外层菌丝），长短不一，直径 3～8（～16）μm，横隔偶见。

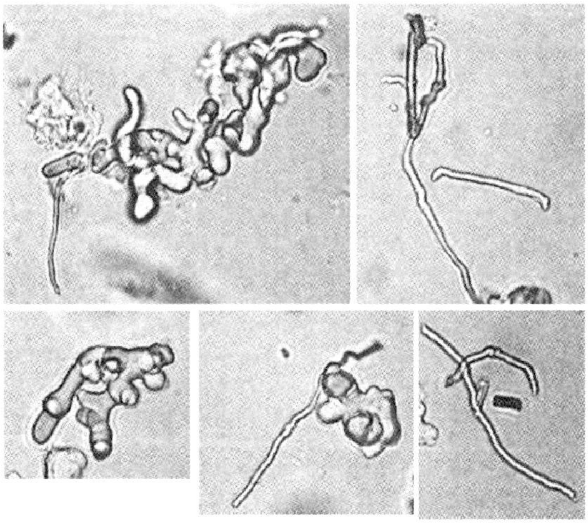

图 8－1　茯苓粉末

3. 理化鉴别

（1）粉末少许加碘化钾碘试液1滴，显深红色；加α－萘酚试液及浓硫酸，显橙红至深红色。

（2）取粉末1 g，加丙酮10 ml，加热回流10分钟，滤过，滤液蒸干，残渣加冰醋酸1 ml使溶解，再加硫酸1滴，显淡红色，后变淡褐色。

（3）薄层层析：取粉末2 g，加乙醚4 ml，冷浸24小时，滤过，滤液浓缩至1 ml，点样于中性氧化铝板上，用苯∶乙醇（9∶1）上行展开，在紫外灯（254 nm）下有黄绿色及紫色两个荧光斑点出现。

【实验作业】

1. 记述茯苓药材性状，包括茯苓个、茯苓皮、茯苓块。
2. 绘茯苓粉末特征图，示菌丝及多糖团块。
3. 记录茯苓理化鉴别实验结果。

【思考题】

1. 茯苓来源于何科属？
2. 茯苓常加工成哪几种商品药材？

8 Identification of Poria (Fungi)

Objectives

1. Master the description and microscopic identification of Poria.
2. Master the physico-chemical identification on Poria.

Experiment Material

Crude drug specimens of Fulingge, Fulingpi and Fulingkuai from *Poria cocos* (Schw.) Wolf and their powder.

Experiment Methods

1. Description

(1) Fulingge: subglobose, ellipsoid or irregular-shaped, variable in size. The outer skin thin and rough, brown to blackish-brown, conspicuously shrivelled and striated, sometimes partly dropped off. Texture hard and compact, fracture granular, near the edge pale red, with smart honeycombing hollows, inner part white, rarely reddish, some showing the penetrating roots of pine in the center. Odour, slight, taste, weak and sticky when chewed.

(2) Fulingpi (pared skin of Poria): irregular pieces, externally brown to blackish-brown, internally white or pale brown, texture relatively loose and soft, slightly elastic.

(3) Fulingkuai (peeled and sliced Poria): occurring in pieces or slices, white, pale red or pale brown, smooth and exquisite.

2. Microscopic identification

Powder of Poria

(1) Slides with glycerol-acetic acid TS: irregular granular masses, branched masses and slender hyphae colourless; dissolved gradually on mounting in chloral hydrate solution, the masses dissolved on heating.

(2) Slides with 5% potassium hydroxide solution: hyphae slender, slightly curved, branched, colourless (inner hyphae) or pale brown (outer hyphae), uneven in size, 3~8 μm (rarely up to 16 μm) in diameter, trabecula occasionally seen.

3. Physico-chemical identification

(1) To a small quantity of powder add 1 drop of iodine potassium idodide TS, a

deep red colour is produced; add α－naphthol TS and sulfuric acid, an orange-red to deep red colour is produced.

(2) To 1 g of the powder add 10 ml of acetone, reflux 10 minutes, filter, evaporate the filtrate to dryness, dissolve the residue in 1 ml of glacial acetic acid, add 1 drop of sulfuric acid, a pale red colour is produced, then turning to pale brown colour.

(3) TLC: To 2 g of the powder, add 4 ml of ether, macerate coolly 24 hours, filter, concentrate the filtrate to 1 ml, apply it to the plate of neutral aluminium oxide, developing in benzene-ethanol (9 : 1), Under ultraviolet light lamp (254 nm), a yellowish-green fluoranthene spot and a purple fluoranthene spot appear.

Laboratory Assignments

1. Record the description of Poria, including Fulingge, Fulingpi, Fulingkuai.
2. Draw the characteristic drawing of the powder of Poria, showing hyphae and polysaccharide masses.
3. Record the results of physico-chemical identification of Poria.

Questions

1. What is the origin of Poria?
2. What commercial drugs are Poria processed to?

实验九　裸子植物生药——麻黄的鉴定

【实验目的】

1. 掌握麻黄类生药的性状及显微主要鉴别特征。
2. 掌握麻黄的理化鉴别方法。
3. 熟悉麻黄含量测定的方法。

【实验材料】

草麻黄 *Ephedra sinica* Stapf，中麻黄 *E. intermedia* Schrenk et C. A. Mey. 和木贼麻黄 *E. equisetina* Bge. 的生药标本；草麻黄茎节间横切片，草麻黄粉末。

【实验方法】

1. 性状鉴别

（1）草麻黄　细长圆柱形，直径 1～2 mm，有时带少量灰棕色木质茎。表面淡绿色至黄绿色，有细纵棱 18～20 条；节明显，节间长 2～6 cm，节上有膜质鳞叶，红棕色，长 3～4 mm，下部约 1/2 合生呈鞘状，上部 2 裂（稀 3 裂），裂片锐三角形，先端灰白色，反曲。体轻，质脆，断面类圆形或扁圆形，略呈纤维性，中心暗红棕色。气微香，味涩、苦。

（2）中麻黄　分枝较多，直径 1.5～3 mm，节间长 2～6 cm，细纵棱 18～28 条。膜质鳞叶长 2～3 mm，裂片 3（稀 2）；断面髓部呈三角状圆形。

（3）木贼麻黄　分枝较多，直径 1～1.5 mm，节间长 1.5～3 cm，有不甚明显的细纵棱 13～14 条。膜质鳞叶长 1～2 mm，裂片 2，短三角形，灰白色，先端多不反曲，基部棕红色至棕黑色。

2. 显微鉴别

（1）茎节间组织横切面

①草麻黄：边缘有波状细棱脊 18～20 条。表皮细胞类方形，外壁厚，被厚的角质层，两棱脊间有下陷气孔；在棱脊内侧有下皮纤维束。皮层宽，有少数纤维散在。中柱鞘纤维束新月形，位于韧皮部外侧。维管束外韧型，8～10 个，形成层环类圆形。木质部类三角形。髓薄壁细胞壁非木化，常含红棕色块状物，偶有环髓纤维。表皮细胞外壁、皮层细胞及纤维壁均可见草酸钙砂晶。

②中麻黄：棱脊 18～28 个；维管束 12～15 个，形成层环类三角形；髓薄壁细胞壁微木化，环髓纤维多。

③木贼麻黄：棱脊 13～14 个；维管束 8～10 个，形成层环类圆形；髓薄壁细胞壁木化，无环髓纤维。

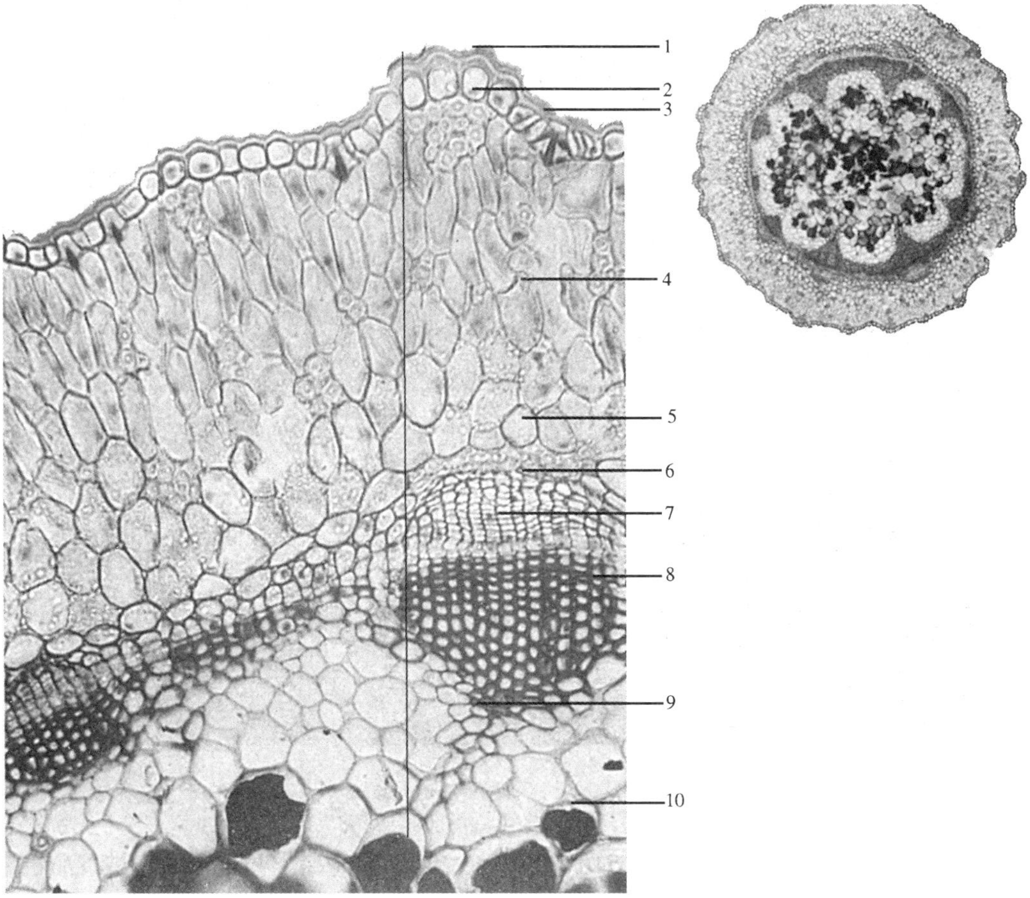

图 9－1　草麻黄茎节间组织横切面

1. 表皮细胞　2. 下皮纤维　3. 气孔　4. 皮层　5. 中柱鞘纤维
6. 韧皮部　7. 形成层　8. 木质部　9. 环髓纤维　10. 髓

（2）草麻黄粉末

①表皮细胞类长方形，外壁布满草酸钙砂晶，角质层厚达 18 μm。

②气孔特异，长圆形，保卫细胞侧面观似电话统状。

③皮层纤维长，直径 10～24 μm，壁厚，有的木化，壁上布满砂晶，形成嵌晶纤维。

3. 理化鉴别

（1）取本品粉末 0.2 g，加水 5 ml 与稀盐酸 1～2 滴，煮沸 2～3 分钟，滤过。滤液置分液漏斗中，加氨试液数滴使呈碱性，再加三氯甲烷 5 ml，振摇提取。分取三氯甲烷液，置两支试管中，一管加氨制氯化铜试液与二硫化碳各 5 滴，振摇，静置，三氯甲烷层显深黄色；另一管为空白，以三氯甲烷 5 滴代替二硫化碳 5 滴，振摇后三氯甲烷层无色或显微黄色。

（2）取本品粉末 1 g，加浓氨试液数滴，再加三氯甲烷 10 ml，加热回流 1 小时，滤过，滤液蒸干，残渣加甲醇 2 ml 充分振摇，滤过，滤液作为供试品溶液。另取盐酸麻黄碱对照品，加甲醇制成每毫升含 1 mg 的溶液，作为对照品溶液。吸取上述两种溶液各 5 μl，分别点于同一硅胶 G 薄层板上，以三氯甲烷－甲醇－浓氨试液（20∶5∶0.5）为展开

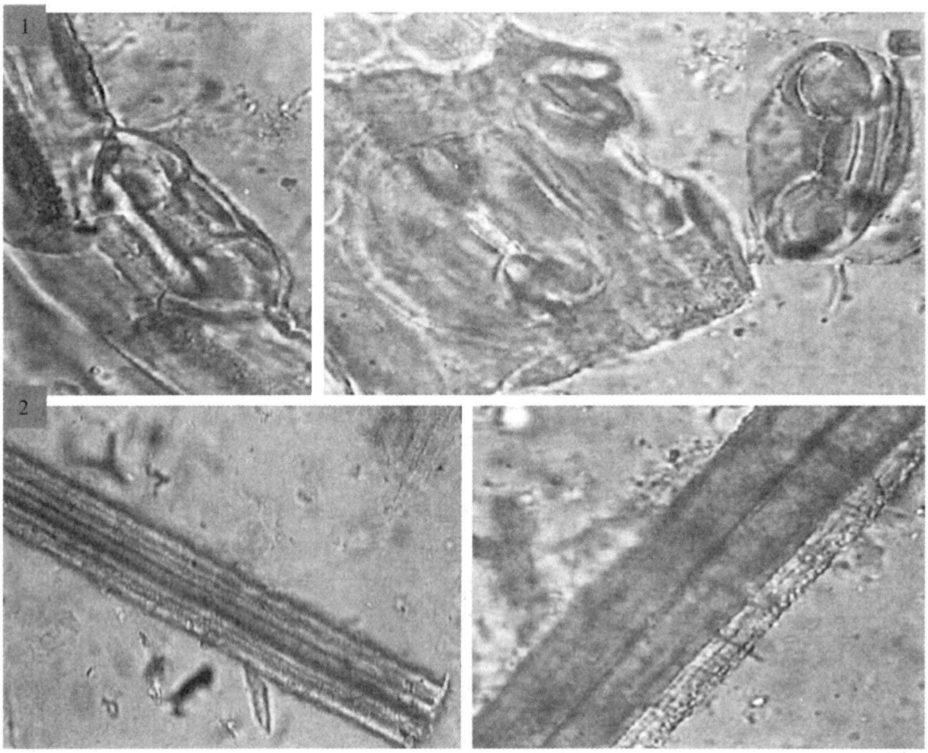

图 9－2　草麻黄粉末

1. 气孔　2. 嵌晶纤维

剂，展开，取出，晾干，喷 2% 茚三酮试液，在 105℃ 加热至斑点显色清晰。供试品色谱在与对照品色谱相应的位置上，显相同的红色斑点。

4. 含量测定

照《中国药典》2005 年版高效液相色谱法测定。

色谱条件与系统适用性试验　以十八烷基硅烷键合硅胶为填充剂；以乙腈－0.1% 磷酸（9:87）为流动相；检测波长为 207 nm。理论板数按盐酸麻黄碱峰计算应不低于 3000。

对照品溶液的制备　精密称取盐酸麻黄碱对照品 10 mg，置 100 ml 量瓶中，用甲醇溶解并稀释至刻度，摇匀。精密量取 2 ml，置 25 ml 量瓶中，用流动相稀释至刻度，摇匀，即得（每 1 ml 含盐酸麻黄碱 8 μg）。

供试品溶液的制备　取本品细粉约 0.2 g，精密称定，置具塞锥形瓶中，精密加入甲醇 25ml，称定重量，超声处理（功率 160 W，频率 50 kHz）45 分钟，放冷，再称定重量，用甲醇补足减失的重量，摇匀，滤过。精密量取续滤液 1ml，置中性氧化铝柱（100～200 目，1.5 g，内径 1 cm）上，用 50% 甲醇洗脱，收集洗脱液约 9 ml，置 10 ml 量瓶中，加磷酸 1 滴，用 50% 甲醇稀释至刻度，摇匀，即得。

测定法　分别精密吸取对照品溶液与供试品溶液各 10～20 μl，注入液相色谱仪，测定，即得。

本品按干燥品计算，含盐酸麻黄碱（$C_{10}H_{15}NO \cdot HCl$）不得少于 1.0%。

【实验作业】

1. 列表记述三种麻黄草质茎横切面的组织特征，并绘草麻黄茎的横切面组织简图。
2. 绘草麻黄粉末特征图，示气孔、嵌晶纤维和导管。
3. 记录理化鉴别各项操作步骤及反应结果，说明其反应原理。

【思考题】

1. 麻黄碱属哪种类型的生物碱？它有哪些理化性质与一般生物碱不一样？
2. 麻黄类药材的原植物，按自然分类法属何种植物，该类植物有何特点？

9 Identification of Herba Ephedrae (Gymnospermae)

Objectives

1. Master the description and microscopic identification of Herba Ephedrae.
2. Master the physico-chemical indentification on Herba Ephedrae.
3. Familiar with the method of determination of Herba Ephedrae.

Experiment Material

Crude drug specimens of *Ephedra sinica* Stapf, *E. intermedia* Schrenk et C. A. Mey. and *E. equisetina* Bge.; Permanent mounts of stem of herb of *E. sinica*; powdered herb of *E. sinica*.

Experiment Methods

1. Description

(1) Herb of *Ephedra sinica* Slenderly cylindrical, 1~2 mm in diameter. Some with a few greyish-brown woody stems. Externally pale green to yellowish-green, with fine longitudinal ridges 18~20. Nodes distinct, internode 2~6 cm long. Scaly leaves on the nodes membranous, reddish-brown, 3~4mm long, about 1/2 base tubularly concrescenced, the upper part with 2 lobes (rarely 3), acutely triangular, apex greyish-white, reversed. Texture light, fragile, fracture, subround or elliptical, slightly fibrous, reddish-brown center. Odour, slightly aromatic; taste, astringent and bitter.

(2) Herb of *Ephedra intermedia* Frequently branched, 1.5~3 mm in diameter. Internode 2~6 cm long, with 18~28 fine longitudinal ridges. Membranous scaly leaves 2~3 mm long, with 3 lobes (rarely 2). Fracture showing a triangular rounded pith.

(3) Herb of *Ephedra equisentina* Frequently branched, 1~1.5 mm in diameter. Internode 1.5~3 cm long, with 13~14 indistinct fine longitudinal ridges. Membranous scaly leaves 1~2 mm long, with 2 lobes, short-triangular, greyish-white, apex infrequently reversed, base brownish-red to brownish-black.

2. Microscopic identification

Transverse section of stem:

(1) Herb of *Ephedra sinica* Waved-shaped fine ridges on fringe 18~20.

Epidermal cells subsquare, covered with thick cuticle, sunken stomata located between two ridges. Hypodermal fibre bundles located in ridges. Cortex broad, a few fibre bundles scattered. Pericycle fibre bundles crescent, outside of phloem. Collateral vascular bundles 8 ~ 10. Cambium ring subround. Xylem subtriangular. Pith parenchymatous cells non-lignified, containing reddish-brown masses; occasionally showing perimedullary fibres. Outer wall of epidermal cells, cortex parenchymatous cells and fibres occurring sandy crystals of calcium oxalate.

(2) Herb of *Ephedra intermedia* ridges 18 ~ 28; vascular bundles 12 ~ 15, cambium ring subtriangular. Pith parenchymatous cells slightly lignified, with numerous perimedullary fibres.

(3) Herb of *Ephedra equisetina* ridges 13 ~ 14; vascular bundles 8 ~ 10, cambium ring subround; Pith parenchymatous lignified, without perimedullary fibres.

Powdered Herb of *Ephedra sinica*

(1) Epidermal cells subsquare, outer wall covered with sandy crystals of calcium Oxalate, cuticle up to 18 μm thick.

(2) Special stoma, long-rounded, phone-like guard cells in side view.

(3) Cortical fibres slender, 10~24 μm in diameter; thickened-walls, sometimes lignified, scatterd with many sandy crystals, formed chimeric fibres.

3. Physico-chemical identification

(1) To 0.2 g of the powder, add 5ml of water and 1~2 drops of dilute hydrochloric acid, boil for 2~3 minutes and filter. Transfer the filtrate to a separator, add several drops of ammonia TS to make alkaline and extract with 5 ml of chloroform. Transfer the chloroform solution into 2 tubes. To one tube add ammoniated cupric chloride TS and carbon disulfide, 5 drops of each, shake well and allow to stand, the chloroform layer becomes deep yellow; to the other tube, add 5 drops of chloroform instead of carbon disulfide as a blank, shake well, the chloroform layer is colorless or slightly yellow.

(2) To 1 g of the powder add several drops of concentrated ammonia TS and 10 ml of chloroform, heat under reflux for 1 hour and filter. Evaporate the filtrate to dryness, add 2 ml of methanol to the residue, mix well, filter, and use the filtrate as the test solution. Dissolve ephedrine hydrochloride CRS add methanol to produce a solution containing 1 mg per ml as the reference solution. Using silica gel G as the coating substance and a mixture of chloroform and methanol and concentrated ammonia TS (20:5: 0.5) as the mobile phase. Apply separately to the plats 5 μl of each of the two solutions, after developing and removal of the plate, dry it in air, spray with 2% ninhydrin TS and heat at 105℃ to the spots clear. The spot in the chromatogram obtained with the test solution corresponds in position and color to the spot in the chromatogram obtained with the reference solution.

4. Assay

Carry out the method for high performance liquid chromatography (Pharmacopoeia of the People's Republic of China, 2005 *ed*).

Chromatography system and system suitability Use octadecylsilane bonded silica gel as the stationary phase and a mixture of acetonitrile and 0.1% phosphoric acid solution (9:87) as the mobile phase. As detector a spectrophotometer set at 207 nm. The number of theoretical plates of the column is not less than 3000, calculated with reference to the peak of ephedrine hydrochloride.

Reference solution Weigh accurately 10 mg of ephedrine hydrochloride CRS to a 100 ml volumetric flask and dilute with methanol to volume. Transfer accurately 2 ml of the solution to a 25 ml volumetric flask, dilute with the mobile phase to volume, mix well as the reference solution (containing 8 μg per ml).

Test solution Weigh accurately 0.2 g of the fine powder to a stopper conical flask, add accurately 25 ml of methanol, weigh, ultrasonic treatment for 45 minutes (power, 160 W; frequency, 50 kHz), allow to cool, weigh again and compensate the loss of the weight with methanol, shake well and filter. Apply accurately 1 ml of the successive filtrate to a small column (a cm in inner diameter) packed with neutral aluminium oxide (100~200 mesh, 1.5 g), elute with 50% methanol. Collect about 9 ml of the elute in a 10 ml volumetric flask, add 1 drop of phosphoric acid, dilute with 50% methanol to volume, mix well.

Procedure Inject accurately 10 ~ 20 μl of the reference solution and the test solution, respectively, into the column, and calculate the content.

It contains not less than 1.0 percent of ephedrine hydrochloride ($C_{10}H_{15}NO \cdot HCl$), calculated with reference to the dried drug.

Laboratory Assignments

1. Make a schedule to record the characters of transverse section of herbaceous stem of three Herba Ephedrae and make a diagrammatic drawing of transverse section of herb of *Ephedra sinica*.

2. Make a diagram of the characters of powdered herb of *Ephedra sinica*, and signify stomata, chimeric fibre and vessel.

3. Note the operating steps and results of physico-chemical identification, explain the mechanism of the reactions.

Questions

1. What type of alkaloid does ephedrine belongs to? What physical and chemical property differ from other alkaloids?

2. What kinds of plants do original plants of Herba Ephedra belong to, according to the natural assorting method? Which characters do these plants possess?

实验十　马兜铃科生药——关木通的鉴定

【实验目的】

1. 掌握关木通的性状、显微的主要鉴别特征。
2. 熟悉关木通的来源及理化鉴别方法。

【实验材料】

东北马兜铃 *Aristolochia manshuriensis* Kom. 的生药标本；关木通茎组织切片及关木通粉末。

【实验方法】

1. 性状鉴别

本品呈长圆柱形，稍扭曲，直径 1～6 cm。表面灰黄色或淡棕黄色，有浅纵沟及棕褐色残余粗皮的斑点。节部稍膨大。体轻，质硬，不易折断，断面黄色或淡黄色，皮部薄，木部宽广，有多层整齐环状排列的导管，射线放射状，髓部不明显。摩擦残余粗皮，有樟脑样臭。气微，味苦。

2. 显微鉴别

（1）茎横切面：最外层有少数木栓细胞残留。栓内层为 20 余列扁平细胞。中柱鞘部位有切向延长的大型纤维束，并有少数石细胞散在。维管束 12 个，外韧型，韧皮部窄，木质部宽广，初生射线较宽而长，次生射线窄而短，使维管束分离成特异的形状（马兜铃科式）。形成层成环。木质部导管大型，直径至 360 μm，多单个散在，切向排列成环，木薄壁细胞稀少，髓窄小。栓内层及射线细胞中有草酸钙簇晶。

（2）粉末淡黄色

①具缘纹孔导管巨大，直径约至 360 μm，多破碎，具缘纹孔椭圆形或类圆形，排列紧密。

②傍管木薄壁细胞类方形或类长方形，壁连珠状增厚，木化，纹孔较密。

③纤维管胞多成束，长梭形，直径 11～20 μm，具缘纹孔口斜裂缝状或十字形。

④石细胞少数，类方形或类长方形，壁较厚，偶或一边薄。

⑤草酸钙簇晶直径约至 40 μm。

3. 理化鉴别

取本品粉末 1 g，加 70％乙醇 20 ml，加热回流 15 分钟，滤过。取滤液点于滤纸上，干后置紫外灯（365 nm）下观察，显天蓝色荧光；于点样处加稀盐酸 1 滴，干后显黄绿色荧光，用氨试液熏后复显天蓝色荧光。

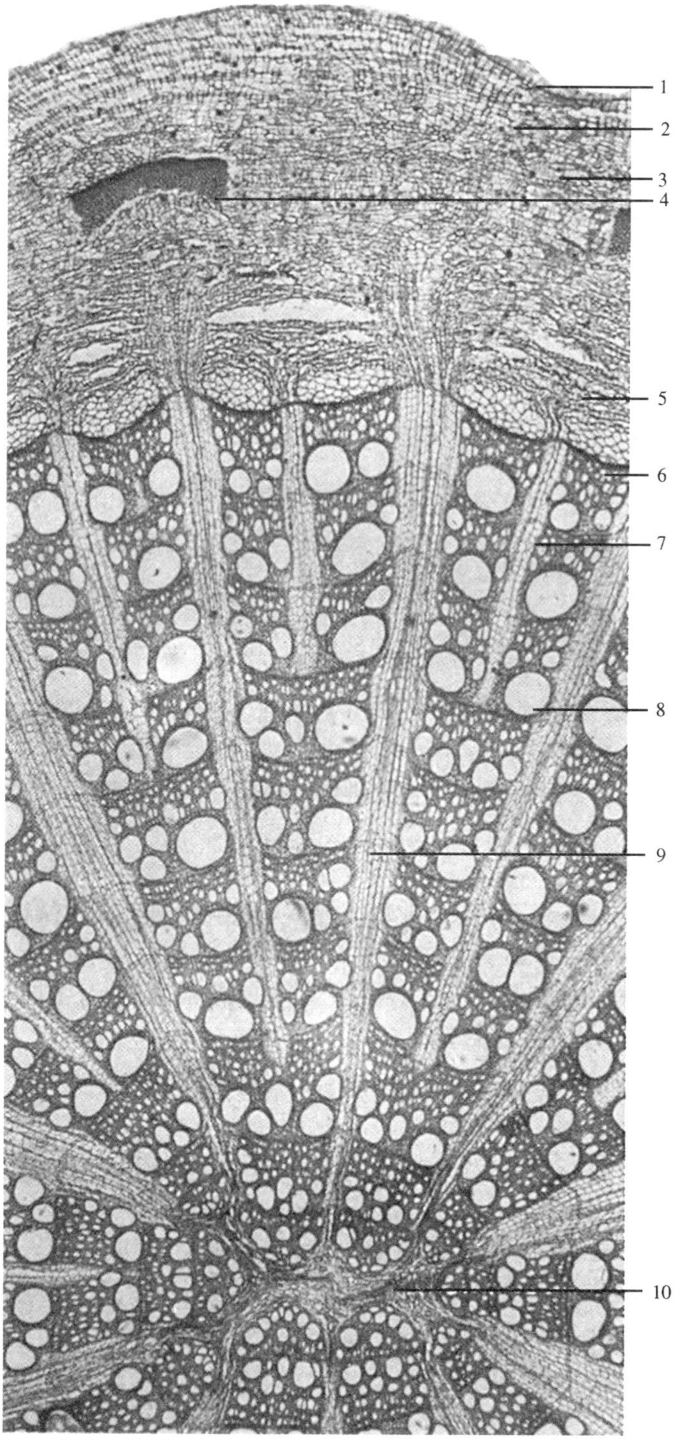

图 10－1　东北马兜铃（茎）横切面

1. 木栓层　2. 栓内层　3. 皮层　4. 中柱鞘纤维　5. 韧皮部　6. 形成层　7. 次生射线　8. 木质部　9. 髓射线　10. 髓

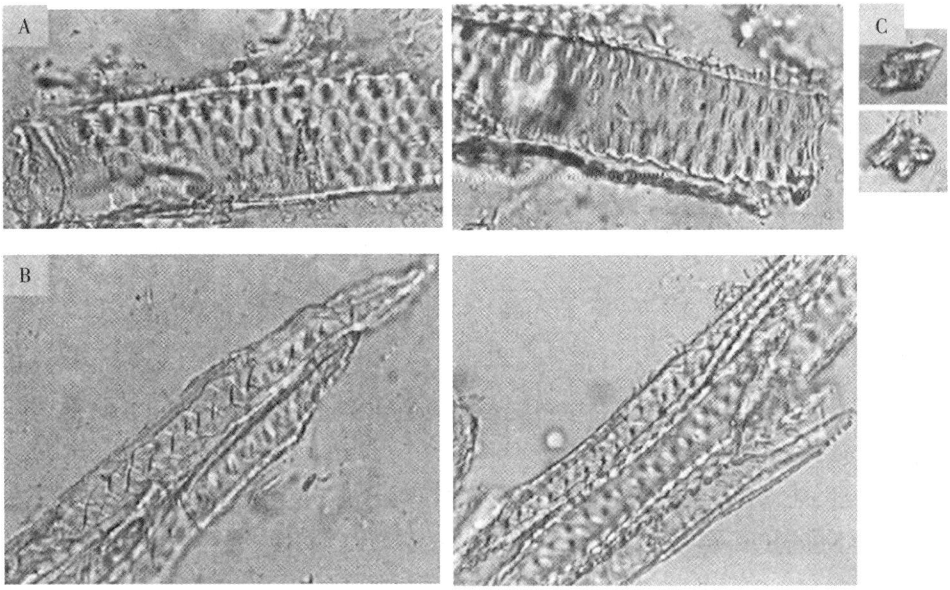

图 10－2　关木通粉末

A. 导管　B. 纤维管胞　C. 草酸钙簇晶

【实验作业】

1. 绘关木通茎横切面组织简图。
2. 绘关木通粉末特征图，示具缘纹孔导管、纤维管胞、傍管木薄壁细胞。
3. 记述关木通理化鉴别步骤与结果。

【思考题】

什么是马兜铃科式维管束？

10 Identification of Caulis Aristolochiae Manshuriensis (Aristolochiaceae)

Objectives

1. Master the description and micro-identification of Caulis Aristolochiae Manshuriensis.

2. Familiar with the origin and physico-chemical identification on Caulis Aristolochiae Manshuriensis.

Experiment Material

Crude drug specimens of *Aristolochia manshuriensis* Kom., permanent mounts of stem of Caulis Aristolochiae Manshuriensis and powered Caulis Aristolochiae Manshuriensis.

Experiment Methods

1. Description

Long cylindrical, slightly twisted, 1~6 cm in diameter. Externally greyish-yellow or brownish-yellow, with shallow longitudinal grooves and adhering remains of brown patches of coarse bark. Nodes slightly swollen. Texture light, compact, uneasily broken, fracture yellow or pale yellow, bark narrow, wood broad and exhibiting vessels arranged in many rings, rays radial, pith indistinct. The drug gives off a smell like camphor on rubbing the remains of coarse bark. Odour, slight; taste, bitter.

2. Microscopic identification

Transverse section of stem: The outset layer with a few cork cells remained. Phelloderm consisting of more than 20 rows of flattened cells. Large fibre bundles in pericycle vertical extended, and a few stone cells scattered in pericycle. Vascular bundles 12, collateral, phloem narrow, xylem wide and broad. Primary rays wider and longer, secondary rays narrower and shorter, which made vascular bundle divided into special shape (Aristolochiaceae vascular bundle). Cambium in ring. Vessels large, up to 360 μm in diameter, single scattered, vertical arranged in a ring. Xylem parenchymatous cells rare. Pith small and narrow. Clusters of calcium oxalate can be seen in phelloderm and ray cells.

Powder: Pale yellow.

(1) Bordered-pitted vessels large, up to 360 μm in diameter, bordered- pit elliptical or subround, arranged closely.

(2) Xylem parenchymatous cells subrectangular or subsquare, walls, walls beaded thickened, lignified. Pit canals relatively close.

(3) Most fibre tracheids in bundles, long fusiform, 11~20 μm in diameter, the pit apertures oblique slit or crossed.

(4) Stone cells infrequent, subsquare or subpolygonal, with relatively thick walls, sometimes thin in one side.

(5) Clusters of calcium oxalate up to 40 μm in diameter.

3. Physico-chemical identification

To 1 g of the powder, add 20 ml of 70% ethanol, heat under reflux for 15 minutes, filter. Spot the filtrate on filter paper, dry it in air, a sky-blue fluorescence is produced under ultra-violet light (365 nm); add 1 drop of dilute hydrochloric acid to the spot, and dry, a yellowish-green fluorescence is shown, which turns to sky-blue fluorescence again on exposing to ammonia TS vapour.

Laboratory Assignments

1. Make a diagnostic drawing of transverse section of Caulis Aristolochiae Manshuriensis.

2. Make a drawing of powder of Caulls Aristolochiae Manshuriensis, and signify bordered-pitted vessels, fiber tracheids and xylem parenchymatous cells.

3. Record the procedure and result of physico-chemical identification of Caulis Aristolochia Manshuriensis.

Questions

What is Aristolochiaceae vascular bundle?

实验十一　蓼科生药——大黄的鉴定与质量标准的制订

【实验目的】

1. 掌握大黄类生药的性状、显微的主要鉴别特征。
2. 掌握大黄的化学成分及理化鉴别方法。
3. 了解大黄质量标准制订方法。

【实验材料】

掌叶大黄 *Rheum palmatum* L.、唐古特大黄 *R. tanguticum* Maxim. ex Balf. 或药用大黄 *R. officinale* Baill. 的生药标本；大黄组织切片及大黄粉末。

【实验内容】

1. 性状鉴别

本品呈圆柱形、圆锥形、卵圆形或不规则块状，长 3～17 cm，直径 3～10 cm。除尽外皮者表面黄棕色或红棕色，有的可见类白色网状纹理及星点（异常维管束）散在，残留的外皮棕褐色，多具绳孔及粗皱纹。质坚实，有的中心稍松软，断面淡红棕色或黄棕色，显颗粒性；根茎髓部宽广，有星点环列或散在；根木部发达，具放射状纹理，形成层环明显，无星点。气清香，味苦而微涩，嚼之粘牙，有砂粒感。

2. 显微鉴别

根茎横切面：木栓层与皮层大多已除去。韧皮部筛管群明显。形成层环明显。木质部射线较密，宽 1～4 列细胞，内含棕色物；导管径向稀疏排列。髓部宽广，其中常见黏液腔，内有红棕色物；异型维管束散在，形成层类圆形，木质部在外，韧皮部在内，射线星芒状。薄壁细胞含草酸钙簇晶，并含多数淀粉粒。

大黄粉末黄棕色。

（1）草酸钙簇晶，直径 20～160 μm，有的至 190 μm。

（2）网纹导管和具缘纹孔导管，非木化。

（3）淀粉粒较多，单粒类球形或多角形，直径 3～44 μm，脐点星状；复粒由 2～8 分粒组成。

3. 理化鉴别

（1）取本品粉末少量进行微量升华，可见黄色菱状或羽状结晶。

（2）本品粉末用 10%硫酸与三氯甲烷提取，三氯甲烷层加氢氧化钠试液，碱液层显红色。

（3）取本品粉末 0.1 g，加甲醇 20 ml，冷浸 1 小时，滤过，取滤液 5 ml，蒸干，残渣加水 10 ml 溶解，滴加盐酸 1 ml，于水浴上加热 30 分钟，立即冷却，用乙醚提取 2 次，每次 20 ml，合并乙醚提取液，蒸干，残渣加三氯甲烷 1 ml 使溶解，作供试品溶液。另取芦荟大黄素、大黄酸、大黄素、大黄酚、大黄素甲醚，加甲醇溶解，使成 1 mg/ml 的溶液，作对照品溶液。吸取上述溶液各 4 μl，分别点于同一以羧甲基纤维素钠为黏合剂的硅

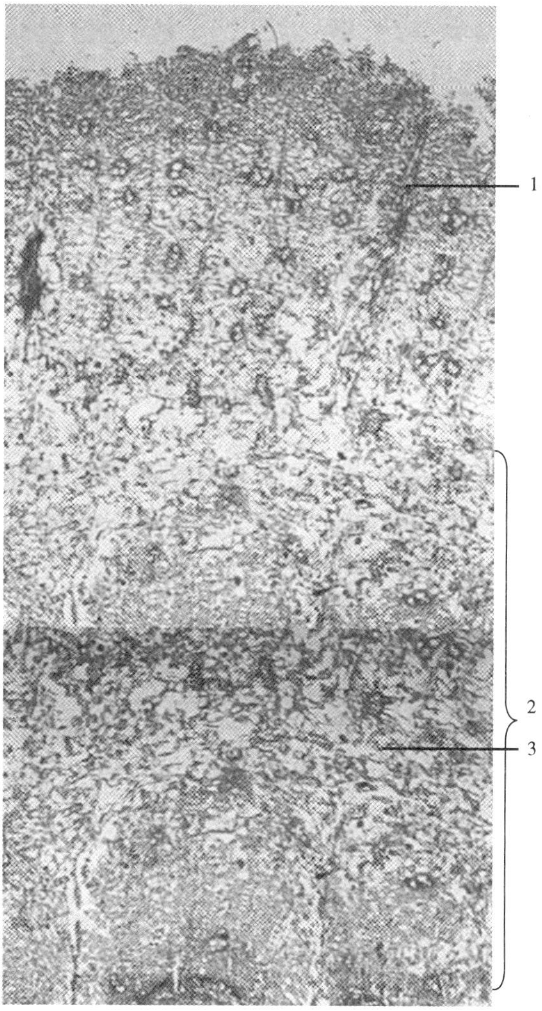

图 11-1　大黄（根茎）横切面
1. 韧皮部　2. 髓　3. 异型维管束

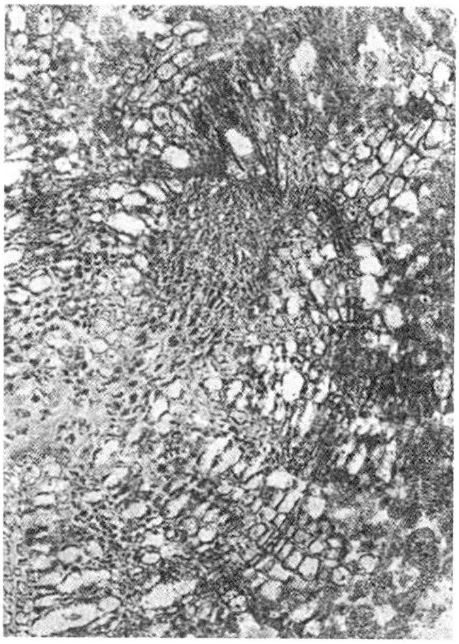

图 11-2　异型维管束

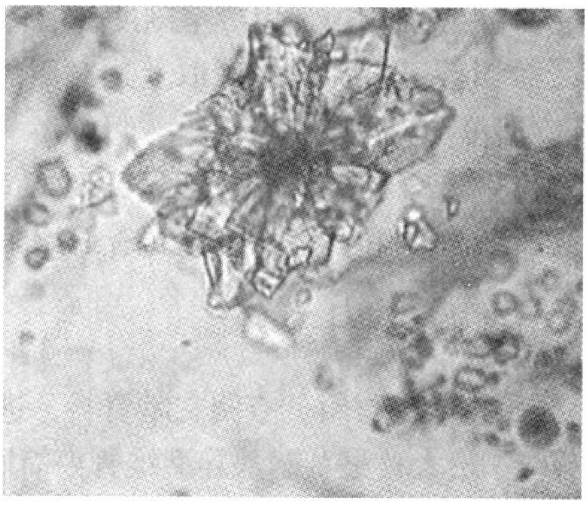

图 11-3　草酸钙簇晶

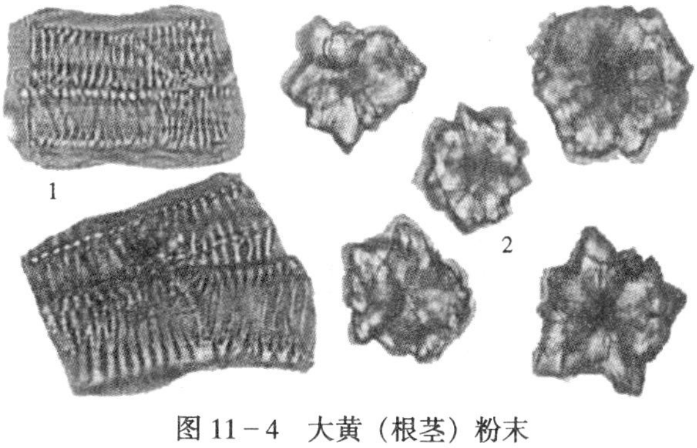

图 11-4　大黄（根茎）粉末
1. 导管　2. 草酸钙簇晶

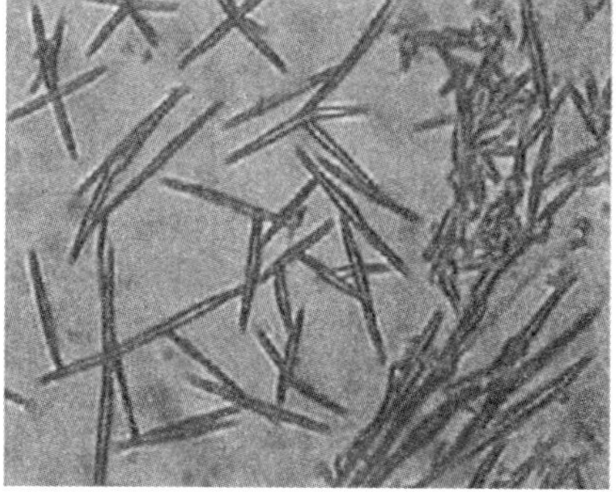

图 11-5　大黄粉末微量升华后结晶

胶H薄层板上，以石油醚（30～60℃）－甲酸乙酯－甲酸（15:5:1）的上层溶液为展开剂，展开，取出，晾干。置紫外光灯（365 nm）下检视，供试品色谱在与对照品色谱相应的位置上显5个相同橙黄色斑点。

4. 含量测定

照《中国药典》2005年版附录高效液相色谱法测定。

色谱条件与系统适用性试验　用十八烷基硅烷键合硅胶为填充剂；甲醇－0.1%磷酸溶液（85:15）为流动相；检测波长为254 nm。理论板数按大黄素峰计算应不低于3000。

对照品溶液的制备　精密称取芦荟大黄素、大黄酸、大黄素、大黄酚、大黄素甲醚对照品适量，加甲醇分别制成每1 ml含芦荟大黄素、大黄酸、大黄素、大黄酚80 μg、大黄素甲醚40 μg的溶液；分别精密称取上述对照品溶液各2 ml，置同一10 ml量瓶中，摇匀，即得（每1 ml中含芦荟大黄素、大黄酸、大黄素、大黄酚各16 μg、含大黄素甲醚8 μg）。

供试品溶液的制备　取本品粉末（过4号筛）约0.15 g，精密称定，置具塞锥形瓶中，精密加入甲醇25 ml，称定重量，加热回流60 min，放冷，再称定重量，用甲醇补足减失的重量，摇匀，滤过，精密称取续滤液5 ml，置烧瓶中，挥去甲醇，加8%盐酸溶液10 ml，超声处理2分钟，再加三氯甲烷10 ml，加热回流1小时，冷却，置分液漏斗中，用少量三氯甲烷洗涤容器，洗液并入分液漏斗中，分取三氯甲烷层，酸液用三氯甲烷提取3次，每次10 ml，合并三氯甲烷液，减压回收三氯甲烷至干，残渣加甲醇使溶解，转移至10 ml量瓶中，加甲醇至刻度，摇匀，滤过，即得。

测定法　分别精密吸取上述对照品溶液与供试品溶液各10 μl，注入液相色谱仪，测定，即得。

本品按干燥品计含芦荟大黄素（$C_{15}H_{10}O_5$）、大黄酸（$C_{15}H_8O_6$）、大黄素（$C_{15}H_{10}O_5$）、大黄酚（$C_{15}H_{10}O_4$）和大黄素甲醚（$C_{16}H_{12}O_5$）的总量不得少于1.50%。

【实验作业】

根据实验材料，查阅文献资料，进行下列实验：

1. 绘大黄根茎髓部异型维管束简图。
2. 记录大黄的理化鉴别、含量测定方法与结果。
3. 查阅文献资料，记述各种大黄的性状鉴别特征，并根据以上实验及文献资料，起草制定大黄药材的质量标准。

【思考题】

1. 大黄主含何种成分，如何鉴别？
2. 大黄混淆品与正品大黄之间的主要区别特征是什么？
3. 除大黄外，还有什么生药组织中具有异型维管束？在构造上有何不同？

11 Identification of Radix et Rhizoma Rhei (Polygonaceae) and the Stipulation of Drug Standards of Quality Control

Objectives

1. Master the description and microscopic identification of Radix et Rhizoma Rhei.
2. Master the chemical constituents and physico-chemical identification on Radix et Rhizoma Rhei.
3. Study to establish the standards of quality control for Radix et Rhizoma Rhei.

Experiment Material

Crude drug specimens of *Rheum palmatum* L., *R. tanguticum* Maxim. ex Balf. or *R. officinale* Baill.; permanent mounts of Radix et Rhizoma Rhei; powder of Radix et Rhizoma Rhei.

Experiment Methods

1. Description

In cylindrical, conical, ovoid or irregular pieces. 3 ~ 17 cm long, 3 ~ 10 cm in diameter. Externally yellowish-brown to reddish-brown when peeled, sometimes whitish reticulations and scattered star spots (abnormal vascular bundles) visible, occasionally with brownish-black patches of cork, mostly with a hole through which the string passed, and coarse wrinkles. Texture compact, some rather loose and soft in the center, fracture pale orange-red or yellowish-brown, granular; pith of Rhizomes broad, with star spots arranged in a ring or irregularly scattered. Wood of the root well developed, lined radially, cambium ring distinct, without star spots. Odour, delicately aromatic; taste bitter and slightly astringent, sticky and gritty on chewing.

2. Microscopic identification

Transverse section of Rhizoma Rhei: Most cork and cortex removed . Sieve tube groups in phloem distinct. Cambium in a ring, xylem with relatively dense rays, 1 ~ 4 cells wide, containing brown masses in ray cells; vessels loosely arrange radically. Pith broad, usually showing mucilage cavities, containing reddish-brown masses; abnormal vascular bundles scattered, cambium subround, xylem at the outside and phloem at the inside; parenchymatous cells containing clusters of calcium oxalate and abundant starch granules.

Powder : yellowish-brown.

(1) Clusters of calcium oxalate, 20 ~ 160 μm, sometimes up to 190 μm in diameter.

(2) Reticulated and bordered-pitted vessels, unlignified.

(3) Starch grains fairly abundant, single granules subsphaeroidal or polygonal, 3~44 μm in diameter, hilum stellate; compound granules consisting of 2~8 components.

3. Physico-chemical identification

(1) Microsublimtion: The microsublimtion consists of small yellow needles if low heat is employed. Higher temperatures result in more or less feathery forms.

(2) To the powder, extracted with 10% sulfuric acid solution and chloroform, add NaOH solution to the chloroform layer, it turns red.

(3) To 0.1 g of the powder add 20 ml of methanol, soak coldly for 1 h, filter. Evaporate 5 ml filtrate to dryness, dissolve the residue in 10 ml of water, add 1 ml of hydrochloric acid, warm on a water bath for 30 minutes and cool immediately, extract with two 20 ml quantities of ether, combine the ether extracts, evaporate to dryness and dissolve the residue in 1 ml of chloroform as the test solution. Dissolve aloe-emodin, rhein, chrysophanol, emodin and physcion in methanol to produce a solution containing 1mg per ml as the reference solutions. Using silica gel H mixed with sodium carboxymethyl cellulose as the coating substance and the upper layer of a mixture of petrol (30~60℃) and ethyl formate and formic acid (15:5:1) as the mobile phase. Apply separately to the plate 4 μl of each of the above solutions. After developing and removal of the plate, dry it in air and examine under UV light (365 nm). The orange-yellow spots in the chromatogram obtained with the test solution correspond in position and colour to the spots in the chromatogram obtained with the reference solution.

4. Assay

Carry out the method for high performance liquid chromatography (Pharmacopoeia of the People's Republic of China, 2005 *ed*).

Chromatographic system and system suitability: Use octadecylsilane bonded silica gel as the stationary phase and a mixture of methanol and 0.1% phosphoric acid (85:15) as the mobile phase. As detector a spectrophotometer set at 254 nm. The number of theoretical plates of the column is not less than 3000, calculated with the reference to the peak of emodin.

Reference solution: Weigh accurately a quantity of aloe-emodin CRS, rhein CRS, emodin CRS, chrysophanol CRS and physcion CRS, respectively, dissolve in methanol to produce five solutions containing 80 μg of each of aloe-emodin, rhein, emodin, chrysophanol per ml and 40 μg of physcion per ml. Measure accurately 2 ml of each above solutions to produce a mixture containing 16 μg of each of aloe-emodin, rhein, emodin, chrysophanol per ml and 8 μg of physcion per ml.

Test solution: Weigh accurately 0.15 g of the powder (through NO.4 sieve) to a stopper conical flask, accurately add 25 ml of methanol and weigh. Heat under reflux for 1 hour, cool, weigh again, replenish the loss of solvent with methanol, mix well and filter. Measure accurately 5 ml of the successive filtrate in a flask, expel the solvent, add 10 ml of 8% solution of hydrochloric acid, ultrasonic treatment for 2 minutes, add 10 ml of chloroform. Heat under reflux for 1 hour, cool, transfer to a separating funnel, wash the flask with a small quantity of chloroform and combine the washings to the separating funnel. Separate the chloroform layer, extract the acid solution again with three 10 ml quantities of chloroform, combine the chloroform extracts and recover the chloroform in vacuum to dryness. Dissolve the residue in methanol and transfer to a 10 ml volumetric flask, dilute with methanol to volume and mix well.

Procedure: Accurately inject 10 μl of each of the reference solution and the test solution, respectively, into the column, and calculate the content.

It contains not less than 1.5 per cent of the total amount of aloe-emodin ($C_{15}H_{10}O_5$), rhein ($C_{15}H_8O_6$), emodin ($C_{15}H_{10}O_5$), chrysophanol ($C_{15}H_{10}O_4$) and physcion ($C_{16}H_{12}O_5$), calculated with the reference to the dried drug.

Laboratory Assignments

According to experimental materials, research documents and data to do experiment as following.

1. Make a diagnostic of transverse section of a star spot of Radix et Rhizoma Rhei.

2. Record the procedure and result of physico-chemical identification on Radix et Rhizoma Rhei.

3. Research documents and data to record the distinguishing characters of Rheum, and draft the stipulation of the quality standard of Radix et Rhizoma Rhei according to the experiment above and the documents and data.

Questions

1. Which constituents do Radix et Rhizoma Rhei contain chiefly? How to identify?

2. What is the main distinguishable characters between confused Rheum and true Rheum?

3. Do you know which tissues of crude drugs possess abnormal vascular bundles besides Radix et Rhizoma Rhei ? What's the difference on the structure?

实验十二　毛茛科生药——黄连的鉴定

【实验目的】

1. 掌握黄连性状、显微的主要鉴别特征。
2. 掌握黄连的化学成分及理化鉴别方法。
3. 了解同属植物黄连类生药的鉴别特征。

【实验材料】

黄连 *Coptis chinensis* French. （味连）、三角叶黄连 *C. deltoidea* C. Y. Cheng et Hsiao（雅连）或云连 *C. teeta* Wall.（云连）的生药标本。黄连组织切片及黄连粉末。

【实验方法】

1. 性状鉴别

(1) 味连：多集聚成簇，常弯曲，形如鸡爪，单枝根茎长 2～8 cm，直径 0.2～0.8cm。表面灰黄色或黄褐色，粗糙，有不规则结节状隆起、须根及须根残基，有的节间表面平滑如茎杆，习称“过桥”。上部多残留褐色鳞叶，顶端常留有残余的茎或叶柄。质坚硬，折断面不整齐，皮部橙红色或暗棕色，木部鲜黄色或橙黄色，呈放射状排列，髓有时中空。气微，味极苦。

(2) 雅连：多为单枝，略成圆柱形，微弯曲，长 4～8 cm，直径 0.5～1 cm。“过桥”较长。顶端有少许残茎。

(3) 云连：弯曲呈钩状，多为单枝，较细小。

2. 显微鉴别

根茎横切面

(1) 味连：木栓层为数列细胞。皮层较宽；石细胞单个或成群散在。中柱鞘纤维成束，或伴有少量石细胞，均显黄色。维管束外韧型，环列。束间形成层不明显。木质部黄色，均木化，木纤维较发达。髓部由薄壁细胞组成，无石细胞。

(2) 雅连：髓部有石细胞。

(3) 云连：皮层、中柱鞘及髓部均无石细胞。

(4) 黄连粉末

①石细胞　鲜黄色；类圆形、类方形、多角形、类长方形、纺锤形或不规则形；壁厚，有的层纹明显，纹孔细小，孔沟有的分叉；有的石细胞壁较薄，胞腔较大。

②纤维　鲜黄色；韧皮纤维纺锤形或梭形，多成束，有时与石细胞相连结，较粗短，壁厚，胞腔小；木纤维较细长，壁较薄，木化，纹孔稀疏。

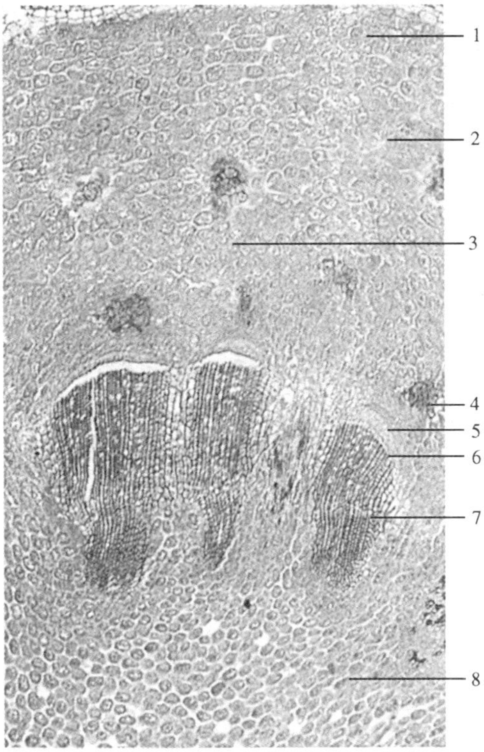

图 12－1 黄连根茎横切面

1. 木栓层 2. 皮层 3. 石细胞 4. 筛管群 5. 韧皮部 6. 形成层 7. 木质部 8. 髓

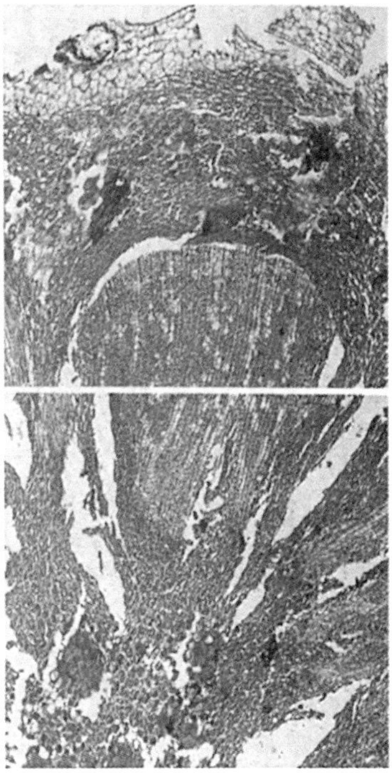

图 12－2 三角叶黄连根茎横切面

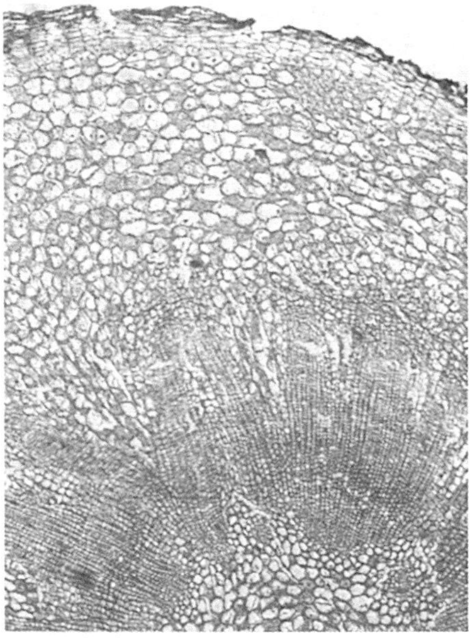

图 12－3 云连根茎横切面

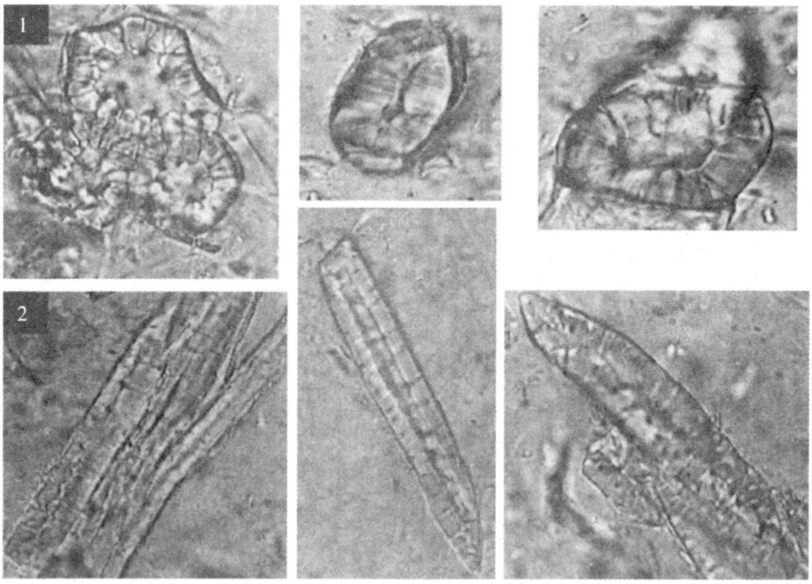

图 12-4　黄连的粉末

1. 石细胞　2. 纤维

3. 理化鉴别

（1）取本品粗粉约 1 g，加乙醇 10 ml，加热至沸腾，放冷，滤过。取滤液 5 滴，加稀盐酸 1 ml 与含氯石灰少量，即显樱红色；另取滤液 5 滴，加 5%没食子酸乙醇溶液 2～3 滴，蒸干，趁热加硫酸数滴，即显深绿色。

（2）取本品粉末 50 mg，加甲醇 5 ml，加热回流 15 分钟，过滤，滤液补加甲醇使成 5 ml，作供试品溶液。另取盐酸小檗碱对照品，加甲醇制成每 1 ml 含 0.5 mg 的溶液，作对照品溶液。吸取上述溶液各 1 μl，分别点于同一硅胶 G 薄层板上，以苯-醋酸乙酯-甲醇-异丙醇-水（6:3:1.5:1.5:0.3）为展开剂，置氨蒸气饱和的展开缸内，展开，取出，晾干，置紫外灯（365 nm）下检视，样品色谱在与小檗碱在相应的位置上显相同的黄色荧光斑点。

4. 含量测定

取本品粉末约 0.1 g，精密称定，置 100 ml 量瓶中，加入盐酸-甲醇（1:100）约 95 ml，60℃水浴上加热 15 分钟，取出，超声处理 30 分钟，室温放置过夜，加甲醇至刻度，摇匀，滤过，滤液作供试品溶液。另取盐酸小檗碱对照品适量，精密称定，加甲醇制成每 1 ml 含 0.04 mg 的溶液，作对照品溶液。照薄层色谱法试验，吸取供试品溶液 1 μl、对照品溶液 1 μl 与 3 μl，交叉点于同一硅胶 G 薄层板上，以苯-醋酸乙酯-异丙醇-甲醇-水（6:3:1.5:1.5:0.3）为展开剂，另槽加入等体积的浓氨试液，预平衡 15 分钟，展开至8 cm,取出，挥干，照薄层色谱法进行荧光扫描，激发波长 $\lambda = 366$ nm，测量供试品与对照品荧光强度的积分值，计算，即得。

本品合小檗碱以盐酸小檗碱（$C_{20}H_{17}NO_4 \cdot HCl$）计，不得少于 3.6%。

【实验作业】

1. 记述三种黄连的性状、组织特征，并绘味连的组织简图。
2. 记录黄连理化鉴别步骤与结果。

【思考题】

三种商品药材（味连、雅连、云连）在来源、产地上有何不同?

12 Identification of Rhizoma Coptidis (Ranunculaceae)

Objectives

1. Master the description and microscopic identification of Rhizoma Coptidis.

2. Master the chemical constituents and physico-chemical identification on Rhizoma Coptidis.

3. Study the characters of different species from Genus *Coptis*.

Experiment Material

Crude drug specimens of *Coptis* chinensis French., *C. deltoidea* C. Y. Cheng et Hsiao or *C. teetta* Wall., permanent mounts of *Coptis* rhizomes, and powered Rhizoma Coptidis.

Experiment Methods

1. Description

Rhizome of *Coptis chinensis*: Mostly gathered to a cluster, curved, like "chicken's feet", single rhizome 2～8 cm long, 2～8 mm in diameter. Externally greyish-yellow or yellowish-brown, rough, bearing irregular nodal protrudings, rootlets and remains of rootlets, some internodes smooth as stem, commonly known as "Guoqiao" (bridge piece). The upper part mostly remained with brown scale leaves, apex often bearing remains of stems or petioles. Texture hard, fracture uneven, bark orange-red or dark brown, wood brightly yellow or orange-yellow, radially arranged, pith sometimes hollowed. Odour, slight; taste, very bitter.

Rhizome of *Coptis deltoidea*: Mostly single, somewhat cylindrical, slightly curved, 4～8 cm long, 0.5～1 cm in diameter. "Guoqiao" relatively long. Apex with some remains of stems.

Rhizome of *Coptis teeta*: Curved hook-like, mostly single relatively small.

2. Microscopic identification

Transverse section:

Rhizome of *Coptis chinensis*: Cork cells of several layers. Cortex broader, stone cells singly scattered or grouped. Pericycle fibres in bundles or accompanied with a few stone cells, both yellow. Collateral vascular bundles arranged in ring. Interfascicular cambium indistinct. Xylem yellow, lignified, xylem fibres well developed. Pith consisting of parenchymatous cells, stone cells absent.

Rhizome of *Coptis deltoidea*: Pith with stone cells.

Rhizome of *Coptis teeta*: Stone cells absent from cortex, pericycle and pith.

Powder:

(1) Stone cells bright yellow, subround, subsquare, subpolygonal, fusiform or irregular, thick-walled, some one with distinct striations, pits small and pit canals crotched, some with relatively thin walls and large lumina.

(2) Fibres bright yellow, phloem fibres long-fusiform or spindle-shaped, mostly in bundles, sometimes connect with stone cells, relatively thick and short, thick-walled, with small lumina. Xylem fibres slender, the walls relatively thin, lignified, pit sparse.

3. Physico-chemical identification

(1) To 1 g of the coarse powder add 10 ml of ethanol, heat to boil, allow to cool, and filter. To 5 drops of the filtrate, add 1 ml of diluted hydrochloric acid and a small quantity of chlorinated lime; a red colour is produced, to another 5 drops of the filtrate add 2 ~ 3 drops of 5% solution of gallic acid in ethanol, evaporate to dryness, and several drops of sulfuric acid to the residue while hot, a dark green colour is produced.

(2) To 50 mg of the powder add 5 ml of methanol, hear under reflux on a water bath for 15 minutes, filter, add methanol to 5 ml used as the test solution. Dissolve berberine hydrochloride CRS in methanol to produce a solution containing 0.5 mg per ml as the reference solution. Using silica gel G as the coating substance and a mixture of benzene, ethyl acetate, methanol, isopropanol and water (6∶ 3∶ 1.5∶ 1.5∶ 0.3) as the mobile phase. Apply separately to the plate 1μl each of the above solutions. After developing in a chamber pre-equilibrated with the vapour of concentrated ammonia TS and removal of the plate, dry it in air and examine under ultra-violet light (365 nm). The yellow fluorescent spot due to berberine hydrochloride in the chromatogram obtained with the reference solution correspond in position and color to the spots in the chromatogram obtained with the test solution.

4. Assay

Weigh accurately 0.1 g of the power to a 100 ml of volumetric flask, add 95 ml of a mixture of hydrochloric acid and methanol (1∶ 100), warm on a water bath (60℃) for 15 minutes, ultrasonic treatment for 30 minutes, allow to stand over night at room temperature, diluted with methanol to the volume, mix well and filter, use the filtrate as the test solutions. Dissolve an appropriate quantity of berberine hydrochloride CRS, accurately weighed, in methanol, to produce a solution containing 0.04 mg per ml as the reference solution. Using silica gel G as the coating substance and a mixture of benzene, ethyl acetate, isopropanol, methanol and water (6∶3∶1.5∶1.5∶0.3) as the mobile phase. Apply 1 μl of the test solution and 1 μl, 3 μl of the reference solution alternatively to the plate. After developing 8cm in a chamber pre-equilibrated with the vapour of concentrated ammonia TS for 15 minutes and removal of the plate, dry it in air. Carry out the method for thin layer chromatography, scan with fluorescence mode at the wavelength of $\lambda_{ex} = 366$ nm, determine the integration value of the fluorescent strength, and calculate the content.

It should contain not less than 3.6% of berberine, calculated as berberine chloride.

Laboratory Assignments

1. Record the characters of description and microscopical identification (Transverse section) of the 3 species from Genus *Coptis*, and make a diagram of transverse section on Rhizome of *Coptis chinensis*.

2. Record the procedure and result of physico-chemical identification of Rhizoma Coptidis.

Questions

What're the differences among three commercial drugs *Coptis chinensis* French., *C. deltoidea* C. Y. Cheng et Hsiao and *C. teeta* Wall. in origin and the producing area?

实验十三　木兰科生药——五味子的鉴定

【实验目的】

1. 掌握五味子性状、显微的主要鉴别特征。
2. 掌握五味子的化学成分及理化鉴别方法。

【实验材料】

五味子 *Schisandra chinensis*（Turcz.）Baill.　（习称“北五味子”）或华中五味子 *S. sphenanthera* Rehd. et Wils.（习称“南五味子”）的生药标本；五味子组织切片及粉末。

【实验方法】

1. 性状鉴别

（1）北五味子：本品呈不规则球形或扁球形，直径5～8 mm。表面紫红色或暗红色，皱缩，显油润；有的表面呈黑红色或出现“白霜”。果肉柔软。种子1～2粒，肾形，表面棕黄色，有光泽，种皮薄而脆。果肉气微，味酸；种子破碎后，有香气，味微咸而辛，微苦。

（2）南五味子：粒较小，表面棕红色或暗棕色，干瘪，皱缩，果肉常紧贴于种子上。

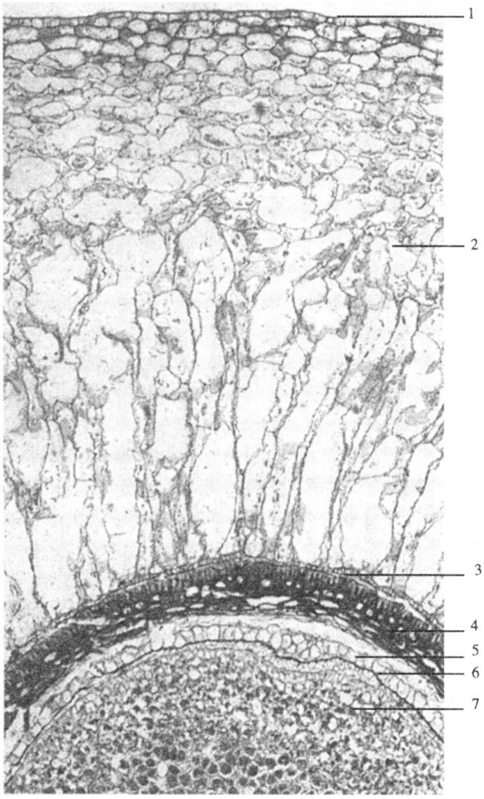

图13－1　五味子果实横切面

1. 外果皮　2. 中果皮　3. 内果皮　4. 种皮石细胞层　5. 油细胞层　6. 种皮内表皮细胞　7. 胚乳细胞

2. 显微鉴别

（1）北五味子果实横切面：外果皮为1列方形或长方形细胞，壁稍厚，外被角质层，散有油细胞；中果皮薄壁细胞十余列，含淀粉粒，散有小型外韧型维管束；内果皮为1列小方形薄壁细胞。种皮最外层为1列径向延长的石细胞，壁厚，纹孔及孔沟细密；其下为数列类圆形、三角形或多角形石细胞，纹孔较大；石细胞层下为数列薄壁细胞，种脊部位有维管束；油细胞层为1列长方形细胞，含棕黄色油滴；再下为3～5列小形细胞；种皮内表皮为1列小细胞，壁稍厚。胚乳细胞含脂肪油滴及糊粉粒。

（2）北五味子粉末暗紫色：种皮表皮石细胞表面观多角形或长多角形，直径 18～48 μm，壁厚，孔沟极细密，胞腔内含深棕色物。种皮内层石细胞呈多角形、类圆形或不规则形，直径约至 83 μm，壁稍厚，纹孔较大。果皮表皮细胞表面观类多角形，角质线纹明显，有类圆形或圆多角形的油细胞散在。中果皮细胞皱缩，含暗棕色物及淀粉粒。

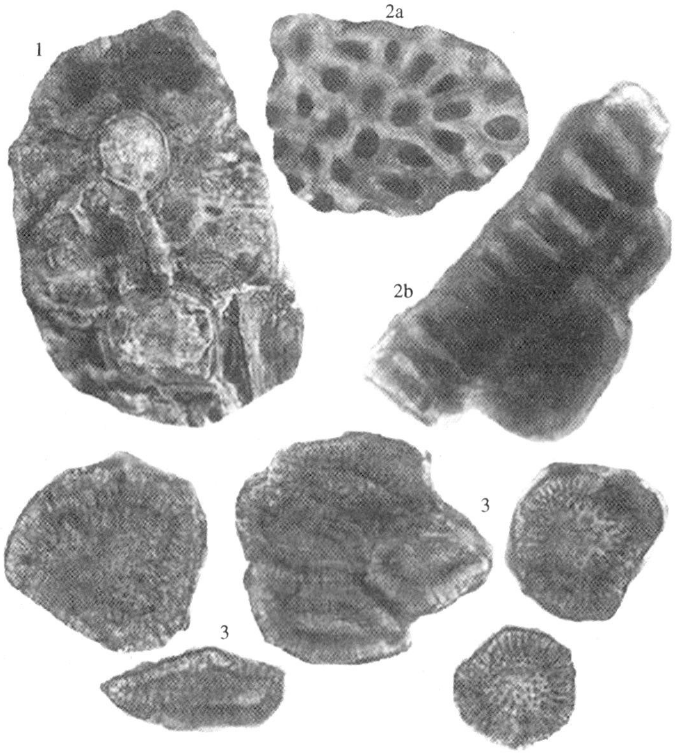

图 13－2　五味子果实粉末

1. 果皮表皮细胞　2. 种皮外层石细胞（a. 表面观　b. 侧面观）　3. 种皮内层石细胞

3. 理化鉴别

（1）取本品粗粉约 1 g，加水 10 ml，浸渍 10 分钟，时时振摇，滤过，滤液浓缩至 2～3 ml，加 5 倍量乙醇，振摇 5 分钟，滤过，滤液挥去乙醇，加水稀释至 10 ml，加活性炭少量，振摇后滤过。取滤液 2 ml，以氢氧化钠试液中和后，加硫酸汞试液 1 滴，煮沸，滤过，滤液加高锰酸钾试液 1 滴，紫红色消失而生成白色沉淀。

（2）取本品粗粉约 1 g，加三氯甲烷 20 ml，加热回流 30 分钟，滤过，滤液蒸干，残渣加三氯甲烷 1 ml 使溶解，作为供试品溶液。另取五味子对照药材 1 g，同法制成对照药材溶液。再取五味子甲素对照品，加三氯甲烷制成每 1 ml 含 1mg 的溶液，作为对照品溶液。吸取上述三种溶液各 2 μl，分别点于同一硅胶 GF_{254}薄层板上，以石油醚（30～60℃）－甲酸乙酯－甲酸（15∶5∶1）的上层溶液为展开剂，展开，取出，晾干，置紫外灯（254 nm）下检视。供试品色谱中，在与对照药材和对照品色谱相应的位置上，显相同颜色的斑点。

【实验作业】

1. 绘五味子果实横切面组织简图。
2. 绘五味子粉末特征图，示种皮石细胞、果皮表皮细胞。
3. 记述五味子理化鉴别步骤与结果。

【思考题】

五味子的主要有效成分是什么?

13 Identification of Fructus Schisandrae (Magnoliaceae)

Objectives

1 Master the description and microscopic identification of Fructus Schisandrae.

2 Master the chemical constituents and physico-chemical identification on Fructus Schisandrae.

Experiment Material

Crude drug specimens of *Schisandra chinensis* (Turcz.) Baill. is known as "Bei Wuweizi" (Northern Magnoliavine Fruit) or *S. sphenanthera* Rehd. et Wils. is known as "Nan Wuweizi" (Southern Magnoliavine Fruit); Permanent mounts of Fructus Schisandrae; powder of Fructus Schisandrae.

Experiment Methods

1. Description

Fruit of *Schisandra chinensis*: Irregularly spheroidal or compressed-spheroidal, 5~8 mm in diameter. Externally red, purplish-red or dull red, shrunken, oily, sometimes externally blackish-red or covered with "white frost". Seeds 1~2, reniform, externally brownish-yellow, lustrous, testa thin and fragile. Odour of pulp, slight; taste, sour. Odour of seeds, aromatic on crushing; taste pungent and slightly bitter.

Fruit of *Schisandra sphenanthera*: Relatively small. Externally brownish-red to dark brown, shrunken and shrivelled, pulp usually adhered to seeds closely.

2. Microscopic identification

Transverse section (*Schisandra chinensis*): Exocarp consisting of 1 layer of square or rectangular epidermal cells, walls relatively thickened, covered with cuticle, oil cells scattered. Mesocarp consisting of 10 or more layers of parenchymatous cells containing starch granules, scattered with small collateral vascular bundles. Endocarp consisting of 1 layer of small square parenchymatous cells. The outermost layer of testa consisting of radially elongated stone cells, thick walled, with fine and dense pits and pit canals; beneath it showing several layers of stone cells, subround, triangular or polygonal with larger pits; underneath the stone cell layers occurring a few layers of parenchymatous cells, vascular bundles occurring in raphes; oil cell layer consisting of 1 layer of rectangular oil cells containing yellowish-brown volatile oil, with 3～5 layers of small cells lying below; inner epidermal cells of testa small, slightly thick-walled; endosperm cells containing oil droplets and aleurone grains.

Powder: Dark purple. Stone cell of epidermis of testa polygonal or elongated-polygonal in surface view, 18～48 μm in diameter, walls thickened with very fine and close pit canals, lumina containing dark brown contents. Stone cells of the inner layers of testa polygonal, subround or irregular, up to 83 μm in diameter, walls slightly thickened, with relatively large pits. Epidermal cells of pericarp polygonal in surface view, with cuticle striations, scattered with oil cells. Cells of mesocarp shrivelled, containing dark brown contents and starch granules.

3. Physico-chemical identification

(1) Add 10 ml of water to 1 g of the coarse powder, macerate for 10 min and shake frequently, filter, concentrate the filtrate to 2～3ml, add 5 folds of ethanol, shake for 5 min, filter and evaporate the alcohol, dilute the residue with 10 ml of water, add a small quantity of decolourizing carbon and filter after shaking. Add sodium hydroxy solution to 2 ml of! the filtrate to make neutral, then add 1 drop of mercuric sulfate, boil, filtes, add a drop of potassium permanganate to the filtrate. The purple colour disappears and a white precipitate is produced.

(2) To 1 g of the powder add 20 ml of chloroform, heat under reflux on a water bath for 30 minutes, filter, evaporate the filtrate to dryness. Dissolve the residue in 1 ml of chloroform as the test solution. Produce a solution of Fructus schisandrae reference drug in the same manner as the reference drug solution. Dissolve deoxyschizandrin CRS in chloroform to produce a solution containing 1 mg per ml as the reference solution. Using silica gel GF_{254} as the coating substance and the upper layer of petroleum ether (30～60℃) -ethyl formate-formic acid (15:5:1) as the mobile phase. Apply separately to the plate 2 μl of each of the three solutions. After developing and removal of the plate, dry it in air, examine under ultraviolet light (254 nm). The spots in the chromatogram obtained with the test solution correspond in position and colour to the spots in the chromatogram obtained with the reference solution.

Laboratory Assignments

1. Make a diagram of the transverse section of Fructus Schisandrae.

2. Make a diagnostic drawing of the powdered Fructus Schisandrae, and signify stone cells, epidermal cells of pericarp.

3. Record the procedure and result of physico-chemical identification on Fructus Schisandrae.

Questions

What are the main active constituents of Fructus Schisandrae?

实验十四　樟科生药——肉桂的鉴定

【实验目的】

1. 掌握肉桂的性状、显微的主要鉴别特征。
2. 掌握肉桂的化学成分及理化鉴别方法。
3. 熟悉皮类生药的鉴别方法。

【实验材料】

肉桂 *Cinnamomum cassia* Presl 的生药标本；肉桂（树皮）组织切片及肉桂（树皮）粉末。

【实验方法】

1. 性状鉴别

本品呈槽状或卷筒状。外表面灰棕色，稍粗糙，有不规则的细皱纹及横向突起的皮孔，有的可见灰白色地衣斑；内表面红棕色，略平坦，有细纵纹，刻划显油痕。质硬而脆，易折断，断面不平坦，外层棕色而较粗糙，内层红棕色而油润，两层间有 1 条黄棕色的线纹。气香浓烈，特异；味甜、辣。

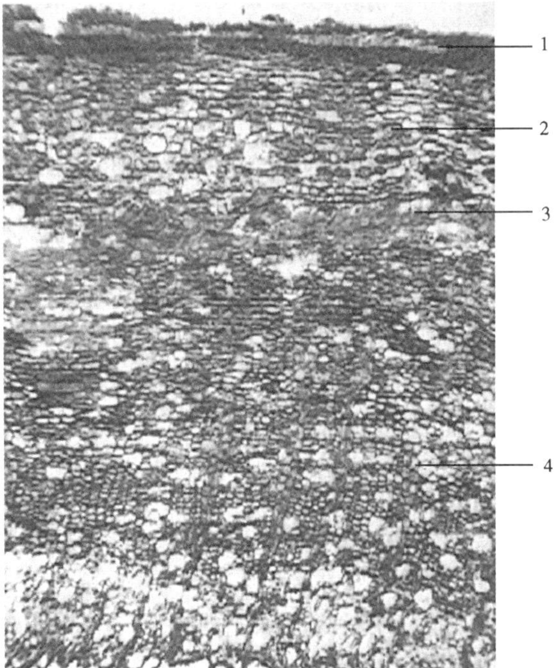

图 14－1　肉桂（树皮）横切面

1. 木栓层　2. 皮层　3. 石细胞群　4. 韧皮部

2. 显微鉴别

（1）组织横切面：木栓细胞数列，最内层细胞外壁增厚，木化。皮层散有石细胞及分泌细胞。中柱鞘部位有石细胞群，断续排列成环，外侧伴有纤维束，石细胞通常外壁较薄。韧皮部射线宽 1～2 列细胞，含细小草酸钙针晶；纤维常 2～3 个成束；油细胞随处可见。薄壁细胞含淀粉粒。

（2）粉末红棕色。

①纤维大多单个散在，呈长梭形，壁极厚，木化。

②石细胞类方形或类圆形，壁厚，有的一面菲薄。

③油细胞类圆形或长圆形。

④草酸钙针晶细小，散在于射线细胞中。

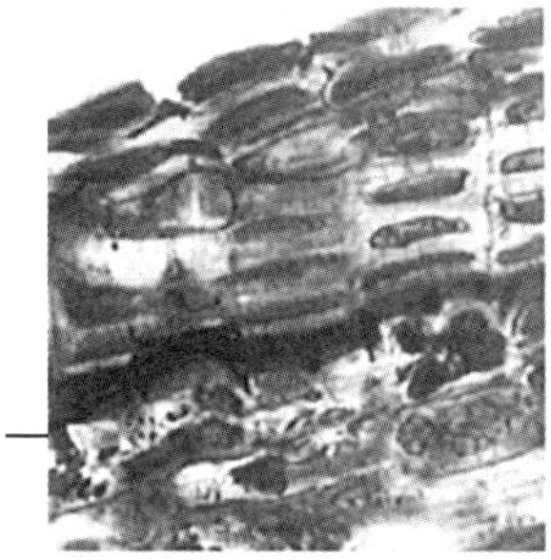

图 14－2　木栓细胞

“→”最内层木栓细胞

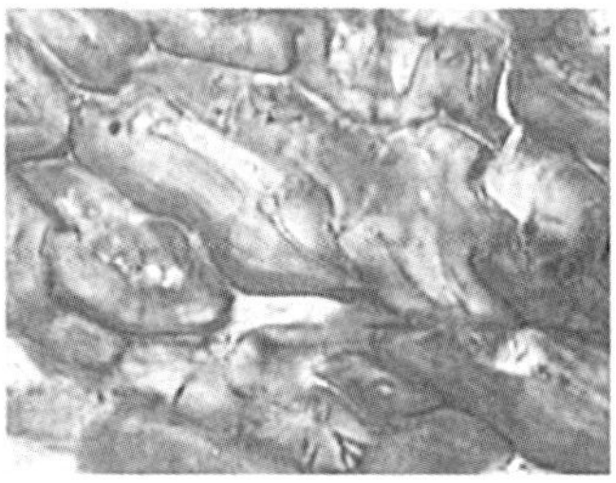

图 14－3　石细胞

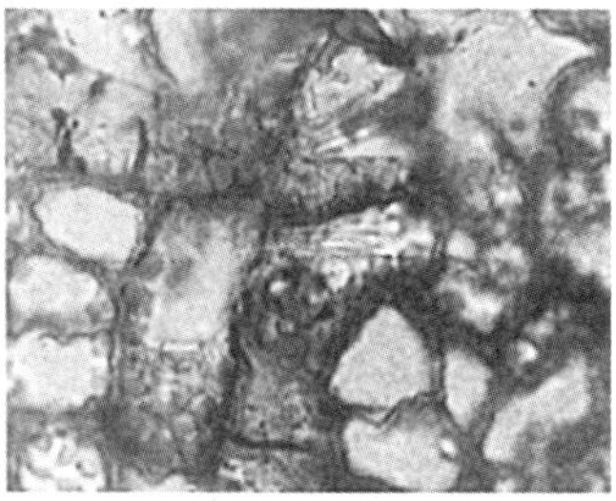

图 14－4　韧皮射线

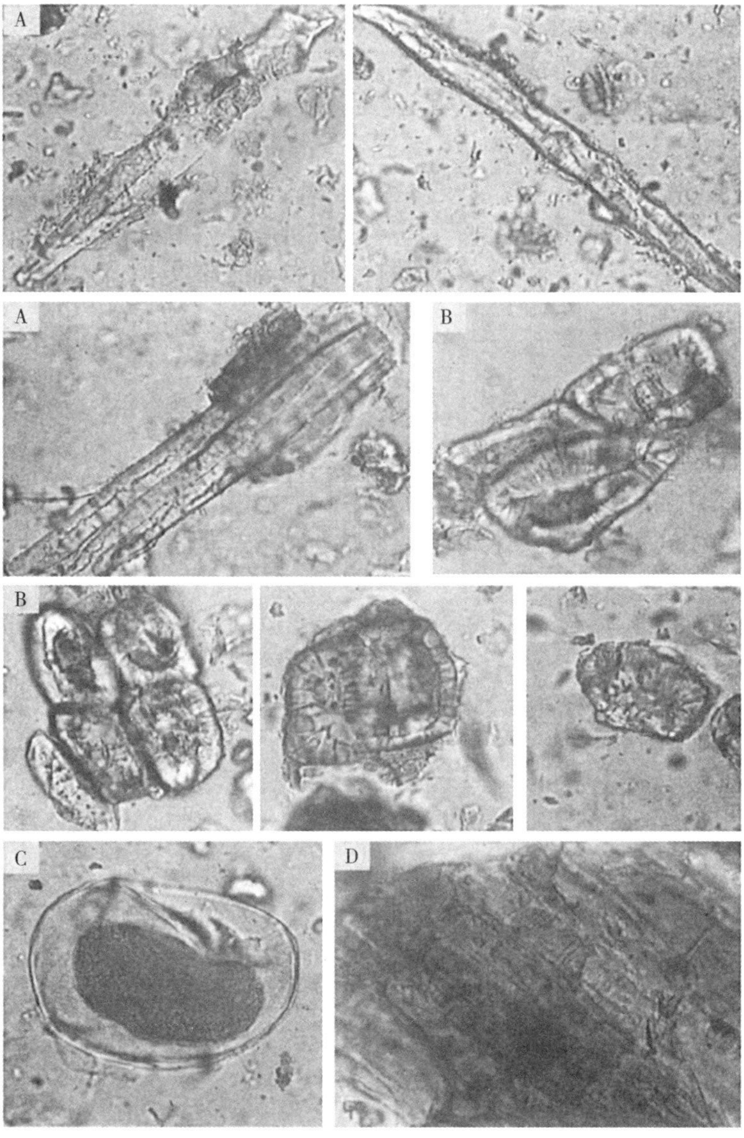

图 14－5　肉桂（树皮）粉末

A. 纤维　B. 石细胞　C. 油细胞　D. 草酸钙针晶（于射线细胞中）

3. 理化鉴别

(1) 取粉末 0.1 g，加三氯甲烷 1 ml 浸渍，吸取三氯甲烷液 2 滴于载玻片上，待挥干，滴加 10%盐酸苯肼试液 1 滴，加盖玻片，镜下可见桂皮醛苯腙杆状结晶。

(2) 取本品粉末 0.5 g，加乙醇 10 ml，密塞，冷浸 20 分钟，时时振摇，滤过，滤液作供试品溶液。另取桂皮醛对照品，加乙醇制成每 1 ml 含 1 μg 的溶液，作对照品溶液。吸取供试品溶液 2～5 μl、对照品溶液 2 μl，分别点样于同一硅胶 G 薄层板上，以石油醚（60～90℃）－乙酸乙酯（17∶3）为展开剂，展开，取出，晾干，喷雾 2，4－二硝基苯肼乙醇试液。供试品在与对照品相对应的位置显相同颜色的斑点。

【实验作业】

1. 绘肉桂横切面组织简图。
2. 绘肉桂粉末特征图，示纤维、石细胞。
3. 记述肉桂理化鉴别步骤与结果。

【思考题】

1. 商品肉桂依采收加工方法不同，可分为哪几种类型？
2. 肉桂的主要成分是什么？显微化学反应所依据的原理是什么？
3. 肉桂与桂皮有何区别？

14 Identification of Cortex Cinnamomi (Lauraceae)

Objectives

1. Master the description and microscopic identification of Cortex Cinnamomi.

2. Master the chemical constituents and physico-chemical identifacation on Cortex Cinnamomi.

3. Familiar with the identification of cortex crude drugs.

Experiment Material

Crude drug specimens of Cortex Cinnamomi, permanent mounts and powder of Cortex Cinnamomi.

Experiment Methods

1. Description

Channelled or quilled. Outer surface greyish-brown, slightly rough, with irregular fine wrinkles and transverse protruding lenticels, some showing greyish-white streaks; inner surface reddish-brown, somewhat even, with fine longitudinal striations and exhibiting oily trace on scratching. Texture hard and fragile, easily broken, fracture uneven, outer layer brown and relatively rough, inner layer reddish-brown and oily, showing a yellowish-brown line between two layers. Odour, strongly aromatic; taste, sweet and pungent.

2. Microscopic identification

Transverse section: Cork cells several layers, the innermost layer of cells with thickened and lignified outer walls. Cortex scattered with stone cells and secretory cells. Pericycle stone cells in groups and arranged in an interrupted ring, accompanied by fibre bundles at outer side, the outer walls of stone cells usually thinner. Phloem rays 1～2 cells wide, containing minute needle crystals of calcium oxalate; fibres usually 2～3 in bundles; oil cells scattered throughout. Parenchymatous cells containing starch granules.

Powder: Reddish-brown.

(1) Most of fibres singly scattered. Long fusiform, walls thickened and lignified.

(2) Stone cells subsquare or subround, walls thickened, some thin at one side.

(3) Oil cells subround or oblong.

(4) Needle crystals minute, scattered in ray cells.

3. Physico-chemical identification

(1) Add 1ml of chloroform to crude drug powder 0.1 g, after digest, imbibe 2 drops of chloroform maceration extract, wait until dry, dropwise a drop of 10% phenylhydrazine hydrochloride, add cover glass, see rhabditiform crystal of cinnamyl aldehyde appear.

(2) Macerate 0.5 g of the powder with 10 ml of ethanol for 20 minutes with frequent shaking in a stoppered flask and filter, use the filtrate as the test solution. Dissolve cinnamic aldehyde CRS in ethanol to produce a solution containing 1 μg per ml as the reference solution. Carry out the method for thin layer chromatography, using silica gel G as the coating substance, and a mixture of petroleum ether (60~90℃) - ethyl acetate (17:3) as the mobile phase. Apply separately to the plate 2~5 μl of the test solution and 2μl of the reference solution. After developing and removal of the plate, dry it in air, spray with ethanolic 2, 4-dinitrophenyhydrazine TS. The spot in the chromatogram obtained with the test solution corresponds in position and colour to the spot in the chromatogram obtained with the reference solution.

Laboratory Assignments

1. Make a diagram of transverse section of Cortex Cinnamomi.

2. Make a diagnostic drawing of powder of Cortex Cinnamomi, and signify fibres, stone cells.

3. Record the procedure and result of physico-chemical identification of Cortex Cinnamomi.

Questions

1. How do we define Cortex Cinnamomi according to its processing and culling?

2. What're the major constituents in Cortex Cinnamomi and the principle of the micro-chemical identification?

3. What's the difference between Cortex Cinnamomi and Cinnamon?

实验十五　十字花科生药——大青叶的鉴定

【实验目的】

1. 掌握大青叶的性状、显微的主要鉴别特征。
2. 了解其他大青叶类生药的植物来源及鉴别特征。

【实验材料】

大青叶（菘蓝 *Isatis indigotica* Fort. 叶）的生药标本和粉末。蓼大青（蓼蓝 *Polygonum tinctorium* Ait. 叶）、马蓝叶（马蓝 *Strobilanthes cusia*（Nees）Bremek 叶）、马大青叶（路边青 *Clerodendron cyrtophyllum* Turcz. 叶）的生药标本。

【实验方法】

1. 性状鉴别

大青叶（菘蓝叶）：叶多卷缩，暗灰绿色，有时破碎仅剩叶柄。完整叶片呈长椭圆形或宽披针形，长 5～20 cm，宽 2～6 cm，先端钝，全缘或微波状，基部狭窄延成翼状叶柄，长 4～10 cm。质脆易碎。气特殊，味微酸、苦涩。

2. 显微鉴别

大青叶粉末绿褐色。

表皮细胞垂周壁较平直或稍弯曲，表面观呈连珠状增厚。下表皮气孔较多，副卫细胞

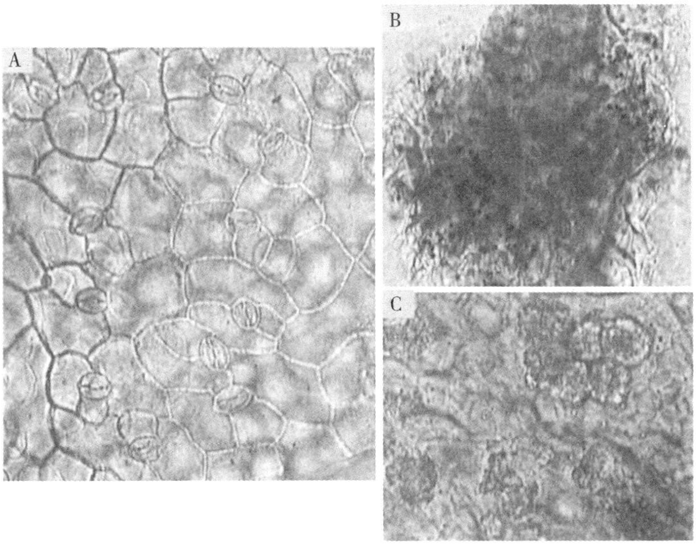

图 15－1　大青叶粉末

A. 表皮细胞和气孔　B. 靛蓝结晶　C. 橙皮苷样结晶

3～4个，不等式，可见2～3个气孔聚集，具共同的副卫细胞。叶肉细胞含靛蓝结晶和橙皮苷样结晶。靛蓝结晶蓝色，呈细小颗粒状或片状，常聚集成堆；橙皮苷样结晶淡黄绿色，呈类圆形或不规则形，有的针簇状。

3. 理化鉴别

取本品粉末0.5 g，加三氯甲烷20 ml，加热回流1小时，滤过，滤液浓缩至1 ml，作供试品溶液。另取靛蓝、靛玉红对照品，加三氯甲烷制成每1 ml各含1 mg的混合溶液，作对照品溶液。吸取上述两种溶液各5 μl，分别点样于同一硅胶G薄层板上，以苯－三氯甲烷－丙酮（5:4:1）为展开剂，展开，取出，晾干。供试品色谱中，在与对照品色谱相应位置上，分别显相同的蓝色斑点和浅紫红色斑点。

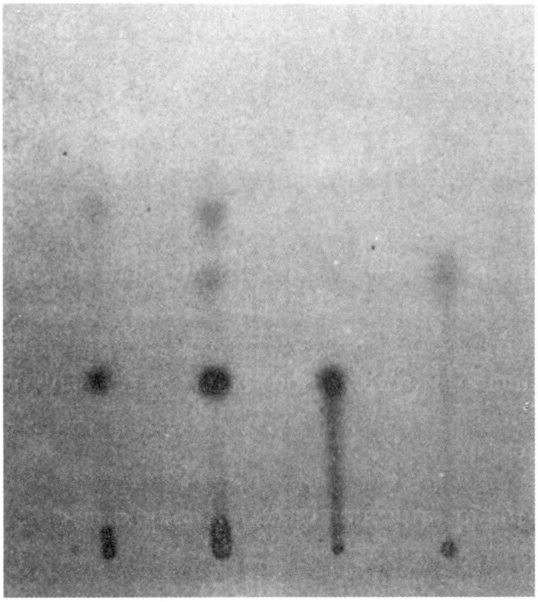

1　　2　　3　　4

图15－2　大青叶薄层层析图谱

1. 商品大青叶　2. 商品大青叶　3. 靛玉红　4. 靛蓝

【实验作业】

1. 绘大青叶叶表皮细胞组织图及气孔图。
2. 记述四种大青叶的鉴别特征。
3. 记述大青叶理化鉴别步骤与结果。

15 Identification of Folium Isatidis (Cruciferae)

Objectives

1. Master the description and microscopic identification of Folium Isatidis.
2. Study the origin and identification of other crude drugs of Folium Isatidis type.

Experiment Material

Crude drug specimens and powder of Folium Isatidis (*Isatis indigotica* Fort.), crude drug specimen of leaves of *Polygonum tinctorium* Ait., *Baphicacanthus cusia* (Nees) Bremek. and *Clerodendron cyrtophyllum* Turcz..

Experiment Methods

1. Description

Folium Isatidis: Mostly crumpled and rolled, sometimes broken, dark greyish-green. When intact, long-elliptical to oblong-oblanceolate, 5~20 cm long, 2~6 cm wide; apex obtuse, margin entire or slightly undulate, base attenuated and decurrent to the petiole appearing wing-shaped; petioles 4~10 cm long. Texture fragile. Odour characteristic; taste slightly sour, bitter and astringent.

2. Microscopic identification

Powder: Greenish-brown. Anticlinal walls of epidermal cells rather straight or slightly sinuous, and beaded in surface view. Stomata anomocytic, with 3~4 subsidiary cells. Indigo-crystals blue, occasionally in small granules or pieces, usually gathered into a pile in mesophyllous cells. Hesperidin-like crystals yellowish-green or colourless, subround or irregular, some ones needle-shaped or clustered, scattered in the mesophyllous cells.

3. Physico-chemical identification

To 0.5 g of the powder add 20 ml of chloroform, heat under reflux for 1 hour, filter and evaporate the filtrate to 1 ml as the test solution. Dissolve indigotin CRS and indirubin CRS in chloroform to produce a mixture containing 1 mg of each per ml as the reference solution. Using silica gel G as the coating substance and a mixture of benzene-chloroform-acetone (5:4:1) as the mobile phase. Apply separately to the plate 5 μl of each of the above two solutions. After developing and removal of the plate, dry it in air. The blue spot and pale purplish-red spot in the chromatogram obtained with the test solution correspond in position and colour to the spots in the chromatogram obtained with the reference solution.

Laboratory Assignments

1. Draw the drafts of leaf's epidermal cells and stomata of Folium Isatidis.

2. Point out the distinguishing characters of four kinds of Folium Isatidis.

3. Record the procedure and result of physico-chemical identification on Folium Isatidis.

实验十六　蔷薇科生药——苦杏仁的鉴定

【实验目的】

1. 掌握苦杏仁性状、显微的主要鉴别特征。
2. 掌握苦杏仁的化学成分及理化鉴别方法。
3. 掌握苦杏仁苷的含量测定方法。

【实验材料】

杏 *Prunus armeniaca* L. 及山杏 *P. armeniaca* L. var. *ansu* Maxim. 的生药标本；苦杏仁粉末。

【实验方法】

1. 性状鉴别

种子呈扁心形，长1～1.9 cm，宽0.8～1.5 cm，厚0.5～0.8 cm。表面黄棕色至红棕色，珠孔位于尖端，近尖端边缘有短线形种脐，钝圆一端较肥厚，有椭圆形合点，种脐与合点间有线形种脊，自合点散出数条深棕色脉纹；种皮与胚乳薄，子叶2枚，肥厚，富油性，胚根介于子叶的尖端部分。气微，与水共研可产生苯甲醛香气；味苦。

2. 显微鉴别

粉末：种皮石细胞单个散在或数个成群，淡黄色或黄棕色。侧面观大多呈贝壳形、类圆形，底部较宽，层纹无或少见，孔沟甚密，上部壁厚5～10 μm，层纹明显，孔沟少；

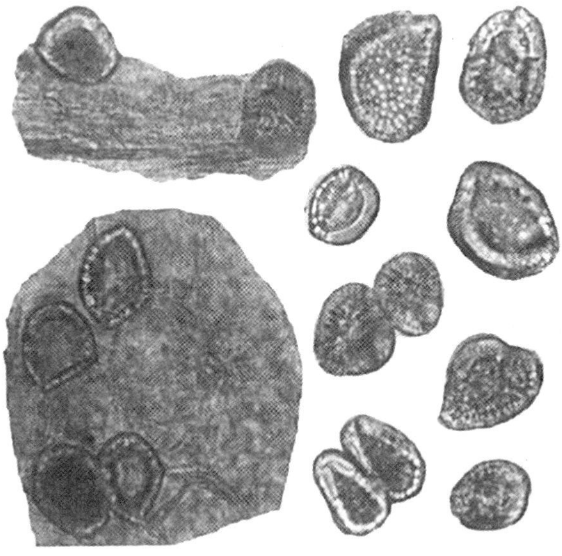

图16－1　苦杏仁（种子）粉末

顶面观呈类圆形、类多角形，纹孔大而密。

S　　1　　2　　3

图 16－2　苦杏仁薄层层析图谱

S. 苦杏仁苷　1. 苦杏仁药材

2. 北杏仁商品　3. 南杏仁商品

3. 理化鉴别

（1）取本品粉末约 1 g，放入试管中，加少许水湿润，试管内悬挂一条苦味酸钠试纸，加塞密闭，将试管置温水浴中，10 分钟后，试纸由黄色转为砖红色。

（2）取本品粉末 1 g，加乙醚 50 ml，加热回流 1 小时，弃去乙醚液，药渣用乙醚 25 ml 洗涤后挥干，加甲醇 30 ml，加热回流 30 分钟，放冷，滤过，滤液作供试品溶液。另取苦杏仁苷对照品，加甲醇制成每 1ml 含 2 mg 的溶液，作对照品溶液。吸取上述两种溶液各 5 μl，分别点于同一硅胶 G 薄层板上，以三氯甲烷－醋酸乙酯－甲醇－水（15∶40∶22∶10）5～10℃ 放置 12 小时的下层溶液为展开剂，展开，取出，立即喷磷钼酸硫酸溶液（磷钼酸 2 g，加水 20 ml 使溶解，再缓缓加入硫酸 30 ml，混匀），105℃ 加热约 10 分钟。供试品色谱中，在与对照品色谱相应位置上，显相同颜色的斑点。

4. 含量测定

取本品粗粉约 15 g，精密称定，置凯氏烧瓶中，加水 150 ml，立即密塞，置 37℃ 水浴中保温 2 小时，连接冷凝管，通水蒸气蒸馏，馏出液导入水 10 ml 与氨试液 2 ml 的吸收液中，接收瓶置冰浴中冷却，至馏出液达 60 ml 时停止蒸馏，馏出液中加碘化钾试液 2 ml，用硝酸银滴定液（0.1 mol/L）缓缓滴定，至溶液显出的黄白色浑浊不消失。每1 ml 硝酸银滴定液（0.1 mol/L）相当于 91.48 mg 的苦杏仁苷（$C_{20}H_{27}NO_{11}$）。

本品含苦杏仁苷（$C_{20}H_{27}NO_{11}$）不得少于 3.0%。

【实验作业】

1. 绘苦杏仁粉末特征图，示种皮石细胞的顶面观与侧面观。
2. 记述苦杏仁理化鉴别的步骤与结果。
3. 记录含量测定结果。

【思考题】

1. 苦杏仁的止咳有效成分是什么？阐明该成分的水解过程。
2. 如何从性状和显微特征上区别山杏仁、杏仁、西伯利亚杏仁和东北杏仁？

16 Identification of Semen Armeniacae Amarum (Rosaceae)

Objectives

1. Master the description and microscopic identification of Semen Armeniacae Amarum.

2. Master the chemical constituents and physico-chemical identification on Semen Armeniacae Amarum.

3. Master the method for determination of amygdalin.

Experiment Material

Crude drug specimens of *Prunus armeniaca* L. or *P. armeniaca* L. var. *ansu* Maxim.; Powdered Semen Armeniacae Amarum.

Experiment Methods

1. Description

Flattened-cordate, 1 ~ 1.9 cm long, 0.8 ~ 1.5 cm wide, 5 ~ 8 mm thick. Externally yellowish-brown to reddish-brown, micropyle situated at the acute end. A short-linear hilum edge of the acute end, rounded end slightly plump, with ellipsoidal chalaza. Line-shaped raphe located between hilum and chalaza, numerous deep-brown veins radiating from chalaza. Testa thin; endosperm thin; cotyledons 2, plump, oily. Radicle located in the acute part of cotyledon. Odour, slightly; grind with water, a characteristic odour of benzaldehyde is perceptible; taste, bitter.

2. Microscopic identification

Powder: stone cells of testa scattered alone or several in groups, pale yellow or yellowish-brown. Almost shell-shaped, subround in section view, slightly wide base, without striation or rarely, colporation dense; the upper wall 5~10 μm thick, striation distinct, rare colporation; subrounded, subpolygonal in surface view, big and dense pit.

3. Physico-chemical identification

(1) Place about 1 g powder into a test tube, moisten with a few water, hang a strip of trinitrophenol TP and stopper tightly. Heat on a warm water bath for 10 minutes, the test paper turns from yellow to a brick red colour.

(2) To 1 g of powder, add 50 ml of ether, heat under reflux for 1 hour, and

discard the ether solution. Wash the residue with 25 ml of ether, then evaporate to dryness, add 30 ml of methanol, and heat under reflux for 30 minutes. Cool to room temperature, filter, and use the filtrate as the test solution. Dissolve a quantity of amygdalin CRS in methanol to produce a solution containing 2 mg per ml as the reference solution. Carry out the method for thin layer chromatography, using silica gel G as the coating substance and the lower layer of chloroform-ethyl acetate-methanol-water (15:40:22:10), on standing at 5～10℃ for 12 hours, as the mobile phase. After developing and removal of the plate, spray immediately with a solution of phosphomolybdic acid in sulfuric acid (to 2 g of phosphomolybdic acid, add 20 ml of water to dissolve, then add slowly 30 ml of sulfuric acid, and mix well), and heat at 105℃ for about 10 minutes. The spot in the chromatogram obtained with the test solution corresponds in position and colour to the spot in the chromatogram obtained with the reference solution.

4. Assay

Place about 15 g of the coarse powder, accurately weighed, in a kjeldahl flask, add 150 ml of water, stopper tightly and immediately, warm on a water bath at 37℃ for 2 hours. Connect the condenser, distill and collect the distillate in a receiver containing 10 ml of water and 2 ml of ammonia TS and cool on an ice bath. Stop the distillation when the distillate is up to 60 ml, add 2 ml of potassium iodide TS to the distillate, and titrate with silver nitrate (0.1 mol/L) VS slowly until a yellowish-white opalescence is produced. Each ml of silver nitrate (0.1 mol/L) VS is equivalent to 91.48 mg of amygdalin ($C_{20}H_{27}NO_{11}$).

It contains not less than 3.0% of amygdalin ($C_{20}H_{27}NO_{11}$).

Laboratory Assignments

1. Make a diagnostic drawing of the powdered Semen Armeniacae Amurum, and signify stone cell of testa in surface view and section view.

2. Record the procedure and result of physico-chemical identification on Semen Armeniacae Amurum.

3. Note the result of determination of amygdalin ($C_{20}H_{77}NO_{11}$).

Questions

1. What is the effective constituents of relieving cough of Semen Armeniacae Amurum? Elucidating the hydrolyzed procedure of this compound.

2. How to identify the seeds of *Prunus armeniaca* L. var. *ansu* Maxim., *P. armeniaca* L., *P. sibirica* L. and *P. mandshurica* (Maxim.) Koehne in description and microscopic characters?

实验十七　豆科生药——甘草的鉴定

【实验目的】

1. 掌握甘草性状、显微的主要鉴别特征。
2. 掌握甘草的化学成分及理化鉴别方法。
3. 了解同属甘草类生药的鉴别特征。

【实验材料】

甘草 *Glycyrrhiza uralensis* Fisch.、胀果甘草 *G. inflata* Bat. 或光果甘果 *G. glabra* L. 的生药标本。甘草 *G. uralensis* Fisch. 根组织切片及粉末。

【实验方法】

1. 性状鉴别

(1) 甘草：根呈圆柱形，长可达 1 m。表面红棕色或灰棕色，具纵皱纹、皮孔及细根痕。质坚硬，折断面粗纤维性。横切面棕色，形成层环明显，射线放射状。根茎表面有芽痕、疤痕，断面中心有髓。气微，味甜而特殊。

(2) 胀果甘草：根及根茎质地粗壮，有的分枝，外皮粗糙，多灰棕色或灰褐色。质坚硬，木质纤维多，粉性小。根茎不定芽多而粗大。

(3) 光果甘果：根及根茎质地较坚实，有的分枝，外皮不粗糙，多灰棕色，皮孔细而不明显。

2. 显微鉴别

(1) 甘草根和根茎横切面：

木栓层为数列棕色细胞。栓内层较窄。韧皮部射线宽广，多弯曲，常现裂隙；纤维成束，非木化或微木化，周围细胞常含草酸钙方晶；筛管群常因压缩而变形。束内形成层明显。木质部射线宽 3～5 列细胞；导管较多，直径约至 160 μm；木纤维成束，周围细胞含草酸钙方晶。根中心无髓；根茎中心有髓。

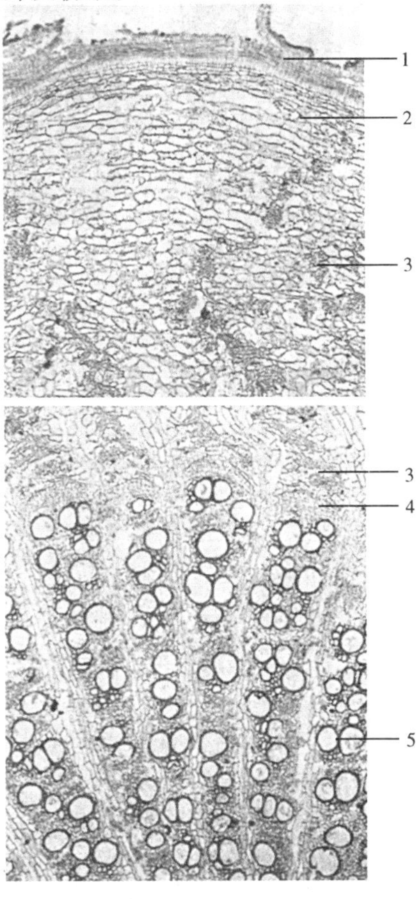

图 17－1　甘草（根）横切面

1. 木栓层　2. 皮层　3. 韧皮部　4. 形成层　5. 木质部（导管）

(2) 粉末淡棕黄色。

①纤维：成束，直径 8～14 μm，壁厚，微木

化，孔沟不明显。晶鞘纤维较多，含晶细胞壁增厚，微木化或非木化。草酸钙方晶呈类双锥形或长方形。

②导管：具缘纹孔导管较大。

③木栓细胞：呈棕红色，壁薄，微木化，表面观呈多角形。

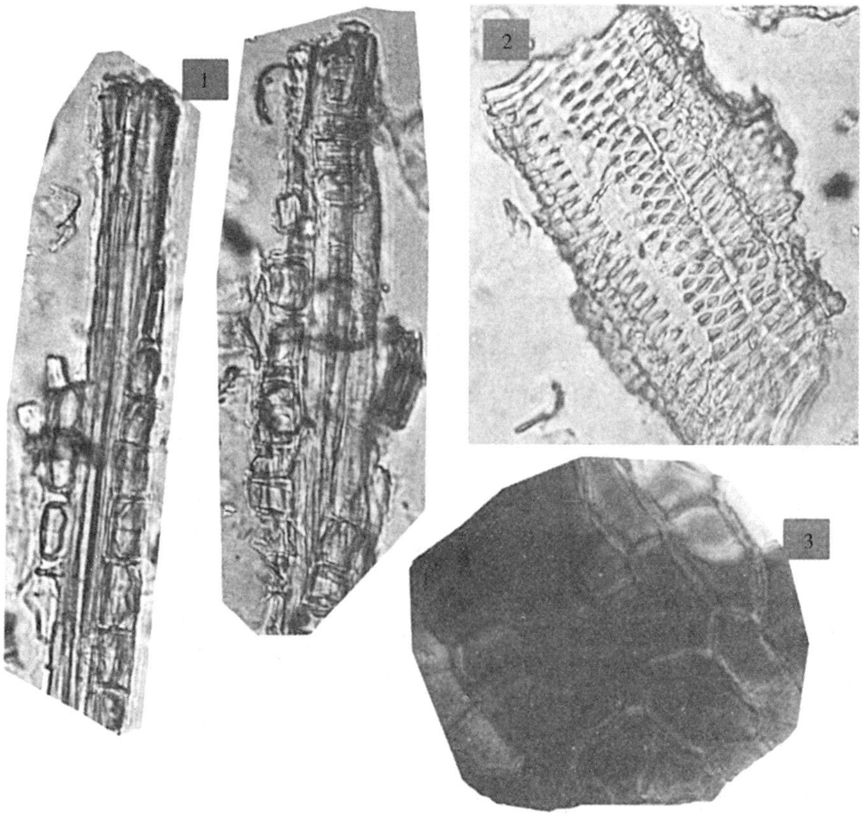

图 17－2　甘草（根）粉末

1. 纤维　2. 导管　3. 木栓细胞

3. 理化鉴别

取本品粉末 1 g，加乙醚 40 ml 加热回流 1 小时，过滤，药渣加甲醇 30 ml，加热回流 1 小时，过滤，滤液蒸干，残渣加水 40 ml 使溶解，用正丁醇提取 3 次，每次 20 ml，合并提取液，用水洗涤 3 次后，蒸干，残渣加甲醇 5 ml 溶解，作供试品溶液。另取甘草对照药材 1 g，同法制成对照药材溶液。再取甘草酸铵对照品，加甲醇制成每 1 ml 含 2 mg 的溶液，作对照品溶液。吸取以上三种溶液各 1～2 μl，分别点样于同一用 1% 氢氧化钠溶液制备的硅胶 G 薄层板上，以醋酸乙酯－甲酸－冰醋酸－水（15∶1∶1∶2）为展开剂，展开，晾干，喷 10% 的硫酸乙醇溶液，105℃加热，在紫外灯（365 nm）下检视，供试品溶液色谱在与对照药材色谱相应的位置上，显相同颜色的荧光斑点；在与对照品溶液色谱的相应位置上，显相同橙黄色荧光斑点。

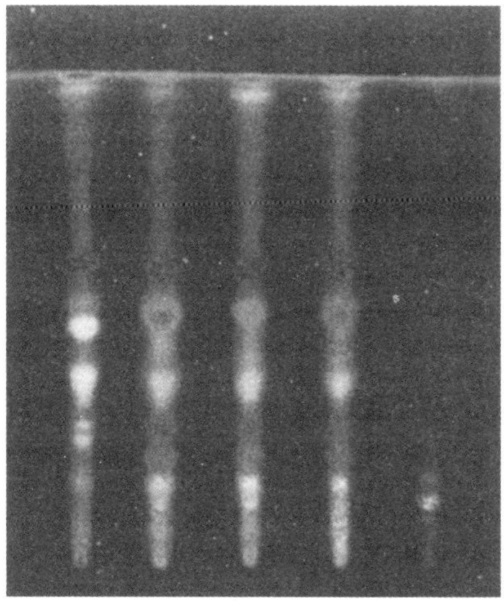

图 17－3　甘草薄层层析图谱

1. 甘草（商品）　2. 甘草（内蒙）　3. 甘草（西北）

4. 甘草（对照药材）　5. 甘草酸（标准品）

【实验作业】

1. 绘甘草根的横切面组织简图。
2. 绘甘草粉末特征图，示晶鞘纤维、导管、木栓细胞。
3. 记述甘草理化鉴别步骤与结果。

【思考题】

1. 什么是晶鞘纤维，它的特点是什么？
2. 甘草的主要成分是什么？
3. 甘草的解毒作用取决于哪一种成分的存在，为什么？

17 Identification of Radix et Rhizoma Glycyrrhizae (Leguminosae)

Objectives

1. Master the description and microscopic identification of Radix et Rhizoma Glycyrrhizae.

2. Master the chemical constituents and physico-chemical identification on Radix et Rhizoma Glycyrrhizae.

3. Study the characters of different species from Genus *Glycyrrhiza*.

Experiment Material

Crude drug specimens of *Glycyrrhiza uralensis* Fisch., *G. inflata* Bat. or *G. glabra* L.; permanent mounts and powder of the root from *G. uralensis*.

Experiment Methods

1. Description

Glycyrrhiza uralensis: Roots cylindrical, 25 ~ 100 cm long, 0.6 ~ 3.5 cm in diameter. The outer bark loose or tight. Externally reddish-brown or greyish-brown, obviously longitudinally wrinkled, furrowed, lenticel-like protruded, and with sparse rootlet scars. Texture compact, fracture slightly fibrous, yellowish-white, starchy, cambium ring distinct, rays radiate, some with clefts. Rizomes cylindrical, externally with bud scars, pith present in the centre of fracture. Odour, slight; taste, sweet and characteristic.

G. inflata: Roots and rhizomes woody and stout, some branched, the outer bark rough, mostly greyish-brown. Texture compact, lignified fibres abundant, and less starchy. Rhizomes with more and large adventitious buds.

G. glabra: Texture of root and rhizomes relatively compact, some branched, the outer bark not rough, mostly greyish-brown, lenticels small and indistinct.

2. Microscopic identification

Transverse section: Cork consisting of several layers of brown cells. Phelloderm relatively narrow. Phloem rays broad, mostly curved, frequently with clefts; most phloem fibres in bundles, unlignified or slightly lignified, surrounded by cells containing prisms of calcium oxalate; sieve tube tissue often pressed to be collapsed. Fascicular cambium distinct. Xylem rays 3～5 cells wide; vessels frequent, up to 160 μm in diameter; xylem fibres in boundles, surrounded by cells containing prisms of calcium oxalate. Roots without pith at the centre; rhizomes possessing pith at the centre.

Powder: Pale brownish-yellow.

(1) Fibres in bundles, slender, 8～14 μm in diameter, thick-walled, slightly lignified, surrounded by parenchymatous cells containing prisms of calcium oxalate, forming crystal fibres. Prisms of calcium oxalate frequent.

(2) Bordered pitted vessels large.

(3) Cork cells reddish-brown, polygonal, slightly lignified.

3. Physico-chemical identification

To 1 g of the powder add 40 ml of ether, heat under reflux on a water bath for 1 hour, filter. Heat the residue under reflux in 30 ml of methanol on a water bath for 1 hour and filter. Evaporate the filtrate to dryness and dissolve the residue in 40 ml of water. Extract 3 times the aqueous solution with three 20 ml quantities of each of *n*-butanol. Combine the *n*-butanol solution wash with water for 3 times and evaporated on a water bath to dryness, dissolve the residue in 5 ml of methanol as the test solution. Prepare a solution of 1 g of Radix et Rhizoma Glycyrrhizae reference drug in the same manner as the reference drug solution. Dissolve ammonium glycyrrhizinate CRS in methanol to produce a solution containing 2 mg per ml as the reference solution. Carry out the method for thin layer chromatography using silica gel G mixed with 1% solution of sodium hydroxide as the coating substance and a mixture of ethyl acetate-formic acid-glacial acetic acid-water (15:1:1:2) as the mobile phase. Apply separately to the plate 1～2 μl of each of the three solutions. After developing and removal of the plate, dry it in air. Spray with 10% solution of sulfuric acid in ethanol. Heat at 105℃ to visualize clearly, and examine under ultraviolet light (365 nm). The fluorescent spots in the chromatogram obtained with test solution correspond in position and colour to the spots obtained with the reference drug solution: an orange fluorescent spot in the chromatogram obtained with the test solution corresponds in position and colour to the spot in the chromatogram obtained with the reference solution.

Laboratory Assignments

1. Make a diagram of the transverse section of *G. uralensis*.

2. Make a diagnostic drawing of the powdered Radix et Rhizoma Glycyrrhizae, and signify crystals fibres, cork cells and vessels.

3. Record the procedure and result of physico-chemical identification of Radix et Rhizoma Glycyrrhizae.

Questions

1. What is crystal fibre? What are its characters?
2. What are the main constituents of Radix et Rhizoma Glycyrrhizae?
3. What is the detoxication constituent of Radix et Rhizoma Glycyrrhizae? Why?

实验十八　豆科生药——番泻叶的鉴定

【实验目的】

1. 掌握番泻叶性状、显微的主要鉴别特征。
2. 掌握番泻叶的理化鉴别方法。

【实验材料】

狭叶番泻叶（*Cassia angustifolia* Vahl 小叶）、尖叶番泻叶（*C. acutifolia* Delile 小叶）的生药标本、叶横切面及粉末。

【实验方法】

1. 性状鉴别

（1）狭叶番泻叶　小叶长卵形或卵状披针形，长 1.5～5 cm，宽 0.4～2 cm，全缘，叶端急尖，叶基稍不对称。上表面黄绿色，下表面浅黄绿色，无毛或近无毛，叶脉稍隆起。革质。气微弱而特异，味微苦，稍有黏性。

（2）尖叶番泻叶　呈广披针形或长卵形，略卷曲，叶端短尖或微突，叶基不对称，两面均有细短毛茸。

2. 显微鉴别

尖叶番泻叶的组织横切面：

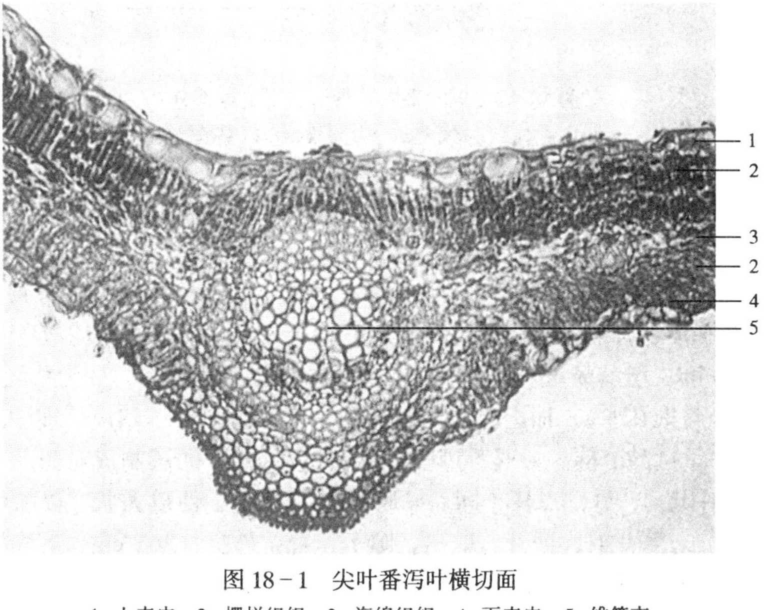

图 18－1　尖叶番泻叶横切面

1. 上表皮　2. 栅栏组织　3. 海绵组织　4. 下表皮　5. 维管束

(1) 上下表皮均有气孔及单细胞非腺毛分布；均有一层表皮细胞，类长方形或类方形，外被角质层，有的表皮细胞含黏液质，黏液积于内壁，占胞腔的1/2以上。

(2) 上下表皮内方均有一列栅栏组织。上表皮下的栅栏组织通过主脉，细胞较长；下表皮内的栅栏组织不通过主脉，细胞较短。

(3) 海绵组织介于上下栅栏组织之间，有的细胞含草酸钙簇晶或方晶。

(4) 主脉维管束外韧型，其上下均有连续的纤维束，纤维束周围细胞有的含草酸钙方晶，形成晶纤维。主脉处的下表皮内有厚角组织。

狭叶番泻叶：与上种近似，仅韧皮部外侧纤维层断续，有的纤维较少。

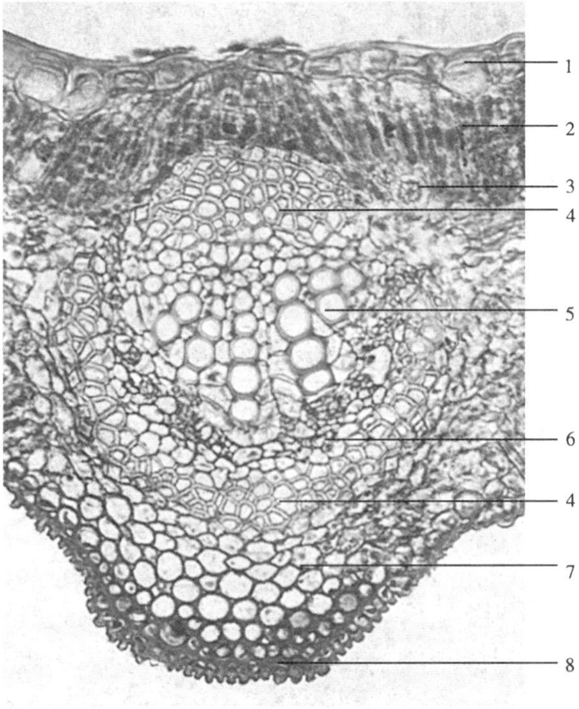

图18-2 尖叶番泻叶横切面（主脉部分）

1. 上表皮 2. 栅栏组织 3. 纤维束 4. 草酸钙簇晶

5. 木质部 6. 韧皮部 7. 厚角组织 8. 下表皮

3. 理化鉴别

(1) 取本品粉末25 mg，加水50 ml及盐酸2 ml，置水浴中加热15分钟，放冷，加乙醚40 ml，振摇提取，分取醚层，通过无水硫酸钠层脱水，滤过，取滤液5 ml，蒸干，放冷，加氨试液5 ml，溶液显黄色或橙色，置水浴中加热2分钟后，变为紫红色。

(2) 取本品粉末0.5 g，加乙醇和水的等量混合溶液3 ml，超声处理30分钟，离心，吸取上清液，作供试品溶液。另取番泻叶对照药材0.5 g，同法制成对照药材溶液。吸取上述两种溶液各10 μl，分别点样于同一硅胶G薄层板上，使成条状，以醋酸乙酯-正丙醇-水（4:4:3）为展开剂，展开，取出，晾干，置紫外灯（365 nm）下检视。供试品色谱中，在与对照药材色谱相应位置上，显相同的颜色的荧光斑点；喷20%硝酸溶液，在

120℃加热约10分钟，放冷，再喷以5%氢氧化钾的稀乙醇溶液，在日光下检视。供试品色谱中，在与对照药材色谱相应位置上，显相同的颜色的斑点。

【实验作业】

1. 绘番泻叶横切面组织简图。
2. 绘番泻叶粉末显微特征图，示晶纤维、非腺毛、表皮细胞及气孔。
3. 记述番泻叶理化鉴别的步骤与结果。

【思考题】

1. 什么是等面叶、异面叶？番泻叶属于哪一类型？
2. 说明番泻叶理化鉴别的原理，所检测的是哪一类成分？

18 Identification of Folium Sennae (Leguminosae)

Objectives

1. Master the description and microscopic identification of Folium Sennae.
2. Master the physico-chemical identification on Folium Sennae.

Experiment Material

Crude drug specimens of *Cassia angustifolia* Vahl and *C. acutifolia* Delile, permanent mounts of Folium Sennae and powdered Folium Sennae.

Experiment Methods

1. Description

(1) Leaf of *Cassia angustifolia*: Elongated ovate or ovate-lanceolate, 1.5～5 cm long, 0.4～2 cm wide, margin entire, apex acute, base slightly asymmetrical. The upper surface yellowish-green, the lower surface pale yellowish-green, glabrous or nearly glabrous, veins slightly prominent. Texture leathery. Odour, slight and characteristic; taste, slightly bitter and mucilaginous.

(2) Leaf of *C. acutifolia*: Lanceolate or elongated ovate, slightly rolled, apex mucronate or slightly convex, base asymmetrical, both surfaces covered with fine, short hairs.

2. Microscopic identification

Transverse section (Leaf of *C. acutifolia*):

(1) Both upper epidermis and lower epidermis bearing stomata, unicellular non-glandular hairs and a row of rectangular or subsquare epidermal cells, covered with cuticle; mucilage gathering to the inner walls of some epidermal cells, occupying 50% of the cells' cavity.

(2) A row of palisade tissue occurring on the inner sides of the upper epidermis and lower epidermis; palisade cells under upper epidermis passing through the main vein, the cells quite long; palisade cells under lower epidermis not passing through the main vein, the cells quite short.

(3) Spongy tissue existing between upper and lower palisade tissues, prisms and clusters of calcium oxalate scattered in some cells.

(4) Vascular bundles of main vein are collateral, both sides of the upper and lower owning continuous fibre bundles. Prisms of calcium oxalate are contained in the cells around fibre bundles, forming crystal fibres. The collenchyma occurring on the inner side of the lower epidermis of main vein.

Leaf of *C. angustifolia*: Be similar to above kind, only the outside of phloem lying intermittently fibre layers, sometimes fibres quite a few.

3. Physico-chemical identification

(1) To 25 mg of the powder add 50 ml of water and 2 ml of hydrochloric acid, heat on a water bath for 15 minutes, allow to cool. Extract with 40 ml of ether, separate the ether layer and dehydrate with anhydrous sodium sulfate and filter. Evaporate 5 ml of the filtrate to dryness, allow to cool, add 5 ml of ammonia TS; a yellow or orange colour is produced, changing to purplish-red when heated on a water bath for 2 minutes.

(2) To 0.5 g of the powder, add 3 ml of a mixture solution of equal quantities of ethanol and water, ultrosonic treatment for 30 minutes, centrifuge. The supernatant is used as the test solution. Prepare a solution with 0.5 g of Folium Sennae reference drug in the same manner as the reference drug solution. Carry out the method for thin layer chromatography, using silica gel G as the coating substance and ethyl acetate-propanol-water (4:4:3) as the mobile phase. Apply separately in strip 10 μl of each of the two solutions to the same plate. After developing and removal of the plate, dry it in air and examine under ultra-violet light (365 nm), the fluorescent spots in the chromatogram obtained with the test solution correspond in position and colour to the spots in the chromatogram obtained with the reference drug solution. Spray with 20% nitric acid solution, heat for 10 minutes at 120℃, allow to cool, spray again with 5% potassium hydroxide solution in dilute ethanol TS, examine in daylight, the spots in the chromatogram obtained with the test solution correspond in position and colour to the spots in the chromatogram obtained with the reference drug solution.

Laboratory Assignments

1. Draw the draft of the transverse section of Folium Sennae.

2. Draw the microscopic distinguishing draft of the powder of Folium Sennae, and signify epidermal cells, stomata, crystal fibres and non-glandular hairs.

3. Narrate the procedure and result of physico-chemical identification about Folium Sennae.

Questions

1. What are the meanings of bifacial leaf and isolateral leaf? Which type does Folium Sennae belong to?

2. Explain the principle of physico-chemical identification on Folium Sennae, point out which kind of constituent can be examined.

实验十九　芸香科生药——黄柏的鉴定与质量标准的制订

【实验目的】

1. 掌握黄柏性状、显微的主要鉴别特征。
2. 掌握黄柏的化学成分及理化鉴别方法。
3. 了解关黄柏与川黄柏的来源及主要区别。

【实验材料】

关黄柏（黄檗 *Phellodendron amurense* Rupr. 树皮）和川黄柏（黄皮树 *P. chinense* Schneid. 树皮）的生药标本；黄柏组织切片及黄柏粉末。

【实验方法】

1. 性状鉴别

(1) 关黄柏　呈板片状或浅槽状，厚 1.5～4 mm。外表面黄绿色或淡棕黄色，较平坦，具有不规则的纵脊和沟纹；内表面黄色或浅黄棕色；体轻，质坚韧，断面纤维性，有的呈裂片状分层，鲜黄色或黄绿色。气微，味极苦，嚼之有黏性。

(2) 川黄柏　厚 1～6 mm。外表黄褐色或黄棕色，平坦或具纵沟纹，有的可见皮孔痕及残存的灰褐色粗皮。内表面暗黄色或淡棕色，具细密的纵棱纹。体轻，质硬，断面纤维性，呈裂片状分层，深黄色。

2. 显微鉴别

(1) 组织横切面

关黄柏　横切面（有残留栓皮）：木栓细胞含黄棕色物。皮层有石细胞和纤维束散在。韧皮部纤维束断续排列成若干层带（硬韧部），与筛管群和韧皮薄壁细胞（软韧部）相间成层排列；纤维众多，纤维束周围细胞含草酸钙方晶形成晶鞘纤维，韧皮射线宽 2～4 列细胞。黏液细胞随处可见。薄壁细胞含草酸钙方晶及淀粉粒。

川黄柏　横切面与关黄柏相似,主要区别为皮层石细胞较多,韧皮部外侧也有少数石细胞。

(2) 关黄柏粉末黄绿色或黄色。纤维鲜黄色，成束散在，周围细胞含草酸钙方晶，形成晶鞘纤维；含晶细胞壁木化增厚。石细胞鲜黄色，类圆形或纺锤形，有的呈分枝状，壁厚，层纹明显。

3. 理化鉴别

(1) 取本品粉末 1 g，加乙醚 10 ml，振摇，过滤，滤液挥干，残渣加冰醋酸 1 ml 使溶解，再加浓硫酸 1 滴，放置，溶液显紫棕色。

(2) 取本品粉末 0.1 g，加甲醇 5 ml，加热回流 15 分钟，滤过，滤液补充甲醇至 5 ml，作供试品溶液。另取黄柏对照药材粉末 0.1 g 同法制成对照药材溶液；再取盐酸小檗碱对照品，加甲醇制成每1ml含0.5 mg的溶液，作对照品溶液。吸取上述三种溶液各1μl，分别点于同一硅胶G薄层板上，以醋酸乙酯-丁酮-甲酸-水（10:6:1:1）为展开剂，置氨蒸气饱和的展开缸内，展开，取出，晾干，置紫外灯（365 nm）下检视。供试品色谱在与对照药材的色谱相对应的位置显相同的荧光斑点；在与对照品色谱相应的位置上，显相同的一个黄色荧光斑点。

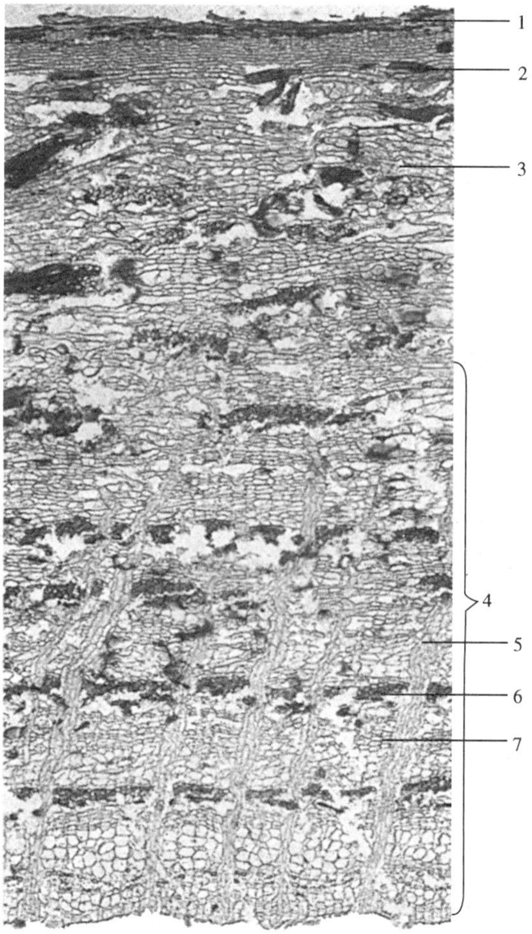

图19-1　关黄柏横切面

1. 木栓层　2. 石细胞群　3. 皮层　4. 韧皮部　5. 射线　6. 硬韧部　7. 软韧部

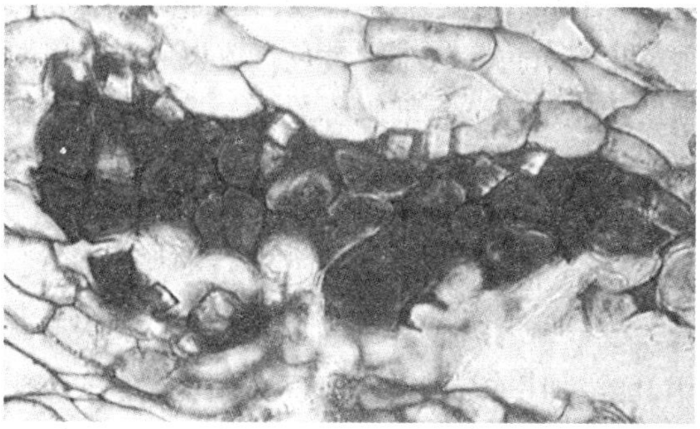

图19-2　纤维束

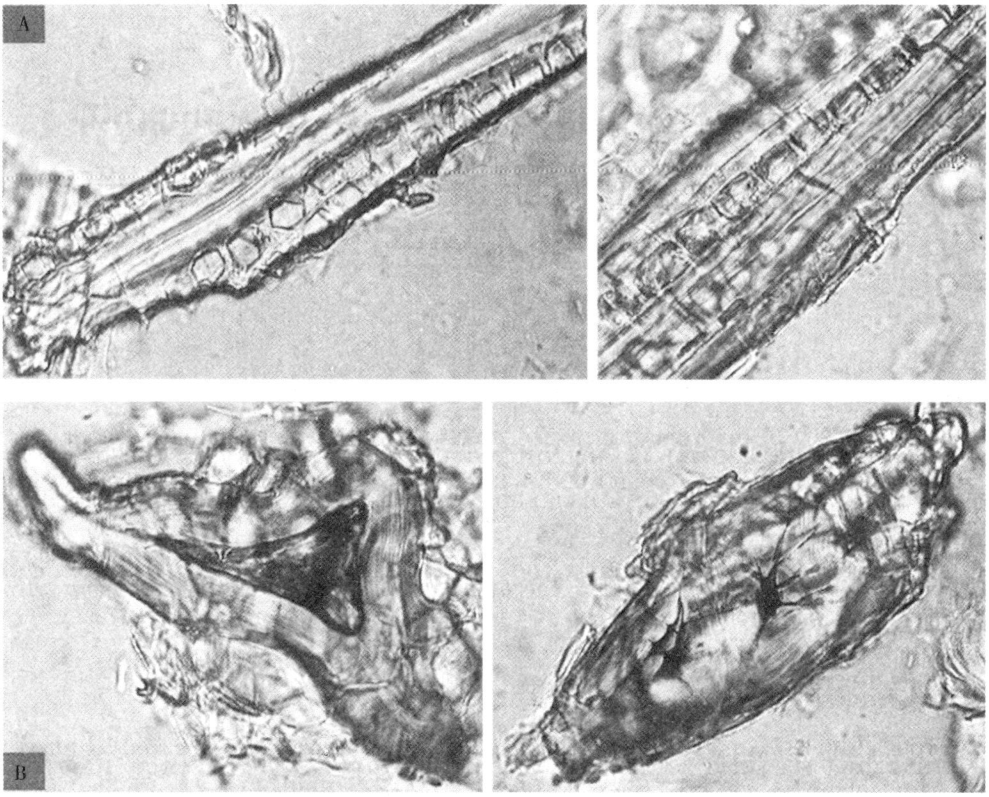

图 19－3　关黄柏粉末

A. 纤维及晶鞘纤维　B. 石细胞

【实验作业】

1. 绘黄柏粉末特征图，示晶鞘纤维、石细胞。

2. 记述黄柏理化鉴别步骤与结果。

3. 查阅文献资料，记述黄柏的性状鉴别、理化鉴别特征，并根据以上实验及文献资料，起草制定黄柏药材的质量标准。

【思考题】

1. 黄柏药材分为川黄柏和关黄柏，两者性状鉴别的主要特征是什么？哪一种质量最佳？

2. 黄柏与黄连均含有小檗碱，如何鉴别它们？

19 Identification of Cortex Phellodendri (Rutaceae) and the Stipulation of Drug Standards of Quality Control

Objectives

1. Master the description and microscopic identification of Cortex Phellodendri.

2. Master the chemical constituents and physico-chemical identification on Cortex Phellodendri.

3. Know about the origin and the main distinction of *Phellodendron chinese* Schneid. and *P. amurense* Rupr.

Experiment Material

Crude drug specimens of Guan huangbo (*Phellodendron amurense* Rupr.) and Chuan huangbo (*P. chinense* Schneid.), permanent mounts of Cortex Phellodendri and powder of Cortex Phellodendri.

Experiment Methods

1. Description

(1) Guan huangbo: Tabular or shallowly channeled, 1.5 ~ 4 mm thick. Outer surface yellowish-green or pale brownish-yellow, relatively even, with irregular longitudinal fissures and longitudinal furrow. Inner surface yellow or pale yellowish-brown. Texture light and relatively hard, fracture fibrous, sometimes showing lobelike layers, bright yellow or yellowish-green. Odour, slight; taste, very bitter, viscous on chewing.

(2) Chuan huangbo: 1 ~ 6 mm thick. Outer surface yellowish-brown, even or longitudinally furrowed, some showing scars of lenticels, and remains of grayish-brown coarse bark, inner surface dark yellow or pale brown, with fine longitudinal ridges. Texture light and hard, fracture fibrous, showing lobelike layers, dark yellow.

2. Microscopic identification

(1) Transverse section

Guan huangbo: Transverse section remains cork, cork cells containing yellowish-brown masses of secretion. Stone cells and fibre bundles scattered in the cortex; fibre bundles of phloem arranging to several layer bands intermittently (hard phloem); fibre bundles putting in order with sieve tubes and parenchymatous cells of phloem (soft phloem) in turn; fibres numerous, prisms of calcium oxalate contained in the cells around fibre bundles, forming crystal fibres; the phloem ray 2～4 rows of cells wide; mucilage cells scattered; parenchymatous cells containing prisms of calcium oxalate and starch grains.

Chuan huangbo: Transverse section similar to Guan huangbo, main difference is that stone cells are quite a few in the cortex and few outside of phloem.

(2) Powder: Greenish-yellow or yellow. Fibres bright yellow, often in bundles, surrounded by parenchymatous cells containing prisms of calcium oxalate, forming crystal fibres; the walls of crystal cells lignified and thickened. Stone cells bright yellow, subbround or fusiform, some branched, walls thickened, with distinct striations.

3. Physico-chemical identification

(1) To 1 g of the powder, add 10 ml of ether, shake well, filter and evaporate the filtrate to dryness. Dissolve the residue in 1 ml of glacial acetic acid, add 1 drop of sulfuric acid and allow to stand; a purplish-brown colour is produced.

(2) Heat under reflux 0.1 g of the powder with 5 ml of methanol for 15 minutes and filter, dilute with methanol to 5 ml as the test solution. Prepare a solution with 0.1 g of Cortex Phellodendri reference drug as the reference drug solution in the same manner. Dissolve berberine hydrochloride CRS in methanol to produce a solution containing 0.5 mg per ml as the reference solution. Carry out the method for thin layer chromatography, using silica G as the coating substance and a mixture of ethyl acetate-butanone-formic acid-water (10∶6∶1∶1) as the mobile phase. Apply separately to the plate 1μl each of the above three solutions. After developing in a chamber saturated with ammonia vapour and removal of the plate, dry it in air and examine under ultraviolet light (365 nm). The fluorescent spots in the chromatogram obtained with the test solution correspond in position and colour to the spots in the chromatogram obtained with the reference drug solution. A yellow fluorescent spot in the chromatogram obtained with the test solution corresponds in position and colour to the spot in the chromatogram obtained with the reference solution.

Laboratory Assignments

1. Draw the characteristic draft of the powder of Cortex Phellodendri, clearly point out the crystal fibres and stone cells.

2. Record the procedure and result of physico-chemical identification about Cortex Phellodendri.

3. Research documents to record the characters of description and physico-chemical identification, and draft the stipulation of the quality standard of Cortex Phellodendri according to the documents and above experiment.

Questions

1. Crude drug of Cortex Phellodendri includes *Phellodendron chinese* Schneid. and *P. amurense* Rupr. Point out their main characters of description and which one has better quality.

2. Both Cortex Phellodendri and Rhizoma Coptidis contain berberine, how to identify them?

实验二十　瑞香科生药——沉香的鉴定

【实验目的】

1. 掌握沉香性状、显微的主要鉴别特征。
2. 掌握沉香的化学成分及理化鉴别方法。
3. 了解不同商品沉香的鉴别特征。

【实验材料】

国产沉香（白木香）*Aquilaria sinensis*（Lour.）Gilg 及沉香 *A. agallocha* Roxb. 的生药标本；国产沉香（白木香）三种切面的组织切片。

【实验方法】

1. 性状鉴别

(1) 国产沉香（白木香）：呈不规则块状、片状或盔帽状，有的为小碎块；表面凹凸不平，有刀痕，偶有孔洞，可见黑褐色树脂与黄白色木部相间的斑纹，孔洞及凹窝表面多呈朽木状。质较坚实，断面刺状。气芳香，味苦。

(2) 进口沉香：呈圆柱形或不规则块片，两端或表面有刀劈痕、沟槽或孔洞，凹凸不平；表面淡黄色或灰黑色，密布断续的棕黑色纵纹（含树脂的木射线），有时可见黑褐色树脂斑痕，微具光泽，横断面可见细密棕黑色斑点。质坚硬而重，能沉或半沉于水。气味较浓烈。

2. 显微鉴别

(1) 国产沉香：横切面　木射线宽 1～2 列细胞，含棕色树脂；导管圆多角形，直径 42～128 μm，有的含棕色树脂；木纤维多角形，直径20～45 μm，壁稍厚，木化；木间韧皮部扁长椭圆形或条带状，常与射线相交，细胞壁薄，内含棕色树脂；其间散有少数纤维。

切向纵切面　射线高 4～15 个细胞；导管具缘纹孔排列紧密；木间韧皮部细胞类长方形。

径向纵切面　射线呈条带状，细胞同型。

(2) 国产沉香粉末

①纤维管胞多成束，长梭形，壁较薄，径向壁上有具缘纹孔。

②导管具缘纹孔排列紧密，内含黄棕色树脂块。

③木射线细胞壁连珠状增厚。

④树脂团块黄棕色。

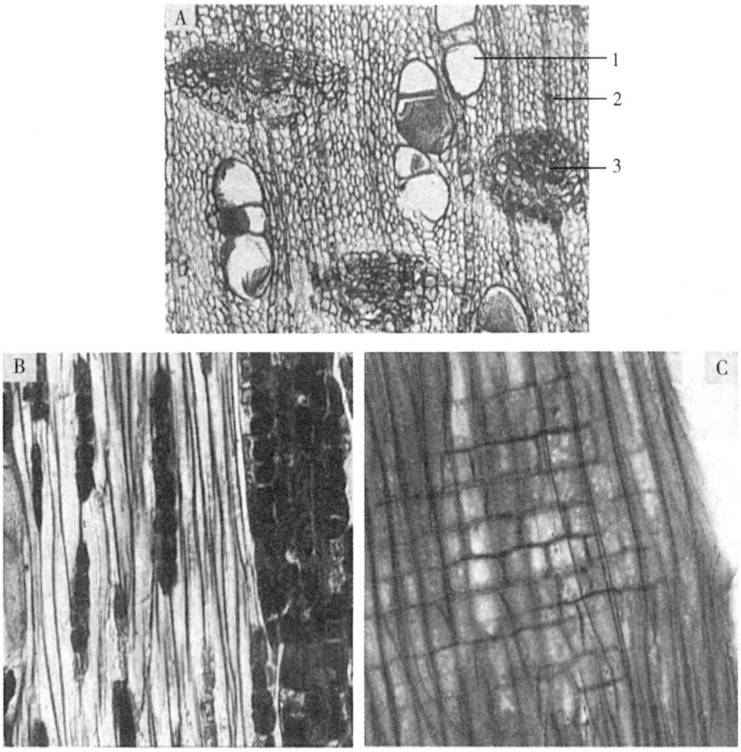

图 20－1　沉香组织三切面
A. 横切面　B. 径向纵切面　C. 切向纵切面
1. 导管　2. 射线　3. 木间韧皮部

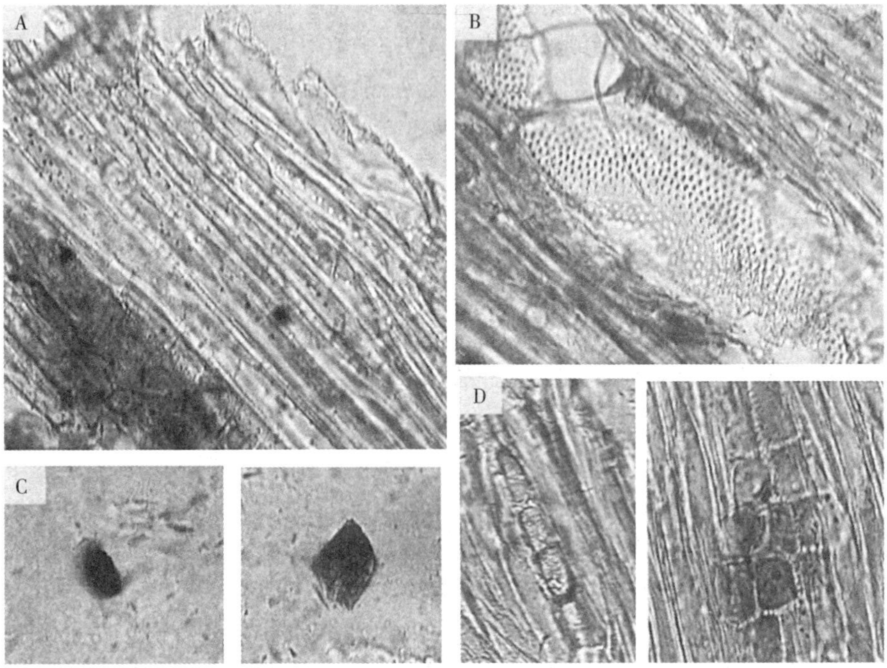

图 20－2　国产沉香粉末
A. 纤维管胞　B. 导管　C. 树脂团块　D. 射线

3. 理化鉴别

取本品粉末约1 g，以乙醇冷浸0.5～1小时，滤过，将滤液蒸干，进行微量升华，得黄褐色油状物，香气浓郁，于油状物上加盐酸1滴与香草醛结晶数粒，再加乙醇1～2滴，渐显樱红色，放置后颜色加深。

【实验作业】

1. 描述国产沉香三个切面组织特征。
2. 记录理化鉴别步骤与结果。

【思考题】

1. 鉴定木类药材三切面时，各切面分别可以观察哪些特征？
2. 进口沉香与国产沉香有何不同？

20 Identification of Lignum Aquilariae Resinatum (Thymelaeaceae)

Objectives

1. Master the description and microscopic identification of Lignum Aquilariae Resinatum.

2. Master the chemical constituents and physico-chemical identification of Lignum Aquilariae Resinatum.

3. Study the characters of different commercial drugs Lignum Aquilariae Resinatum.

Experiment Material

Crude drug specimens of *Aquilariae sinensis* (Lour.) Gilg, *A. agallocha* Roxb., and *Aquilariae sinensis* (Lour.) Gilg's three kinds of tissue section.

Experiment Mathods

1. Description

(1) Chinese eaglewood wood: in irregular lumps and flakes, or helmet-shaped, sometimes in shreds. Externally lumpy, with scars of knife cutting, and showing a few of holes, and streaks formed by black-brown resin alternating with yellowish-white wood. Surface of holes and depressions mostly rottenwood-like. Texture relatively compact, fracture splintery. Odour, aromatic; taste, bitter.

(2) Foreign eaglewood wood: in irregular lumps and flakes or cylindrical. Externally and amphi-lumpy, with scars of knife cutting, furrow, and a few holes, externally black-brown or gray-black, densely covered brown-black longitudinal striation interruptly, and scars of black-brown resin, with burnish slightly, meticulous brown-black spot in transection. Texture relatively pachy and heavy, sagging or floating in water. Odour, relatively intensity.

2. Microscopic identification

Transverse section: Xylem rays 1～2 cells wide, filled with brown resin. Vessels round-polygonal, 42～128 μm in diameter, someone containing brown resin. Xylem fibres polygonal, 20～45 μm in diameter, with slightly thickened and lignified walls.

Interxylary phloem elongated-elliptical or strip-shaped, usually intersecting with rays, and the cells with thin walls, containing brown resin, a few of fibres scattered.

Vertical longitudinal section: ray long about 4 ~ 15 cells, vessels' pits arranged tightly; liber cells rectangel similarity.

Radial longitudinal section: ray strip-shaped, cells homeotype.

Powder:

(1) Fibre tracheid fasciculation mostly, fusiform shape, wall usually thinner, with pit in radial wall.

(2) Vessels' pits arranged tightly, and yellowish-brown resin lump.

(3) Xylem rays cells wall beaded thickening.

(4) Resin mass yellowish-brown.

3. Physico-chemical identification

To 1 g of the powder add ethanol quench for 0.5 ~ 1 hour, filter and evaporate the filtrate to dryness. Microsublime the ethanol-soluble extractives obtained, a yellowish-brown oily substance with strongly aromatic odour is produced. To the oily substance add 1 drop of hydrochloric acid, a small quantity of vanillin and 1 ~ 2 drops of ethanol, a cherry-red colour is gradually produced, and darkens on standing.

Laboratory Assignments

1. Record the characters of three issue sections of *Aquilaria sinensis* (Lour.) Gilg.

2. Record the procedure and result of physico-chemical identification.

Questions

1. What characters can be seen in the three sections of Lignum identification?

2. What are the differences between foreign eaglewood wood and Chinese eaglewood wood?

实验二十一 五加科生药——人参的鉴定

【实验目的】

1. 掌握人参性状、显微的主要鉴别特征。
2. 掌握人参的化学成分及理化鉴别方法。
3. 了解人参类生药的生物技术鉴别方法。
4. 了解人参与西洋参的鉴别特征。
5. 了解常见的人参伪品与人参在性状和显微特征方面的主要鉴别点。

【实验材料】

人参 *Panax ginseng* C. A. Mey. 的生药标本（生晒参、红参）；人参根组织切片及人参粉末。西洋参 *P. quinquefolium* L. 的生药标本。

【实验方法】

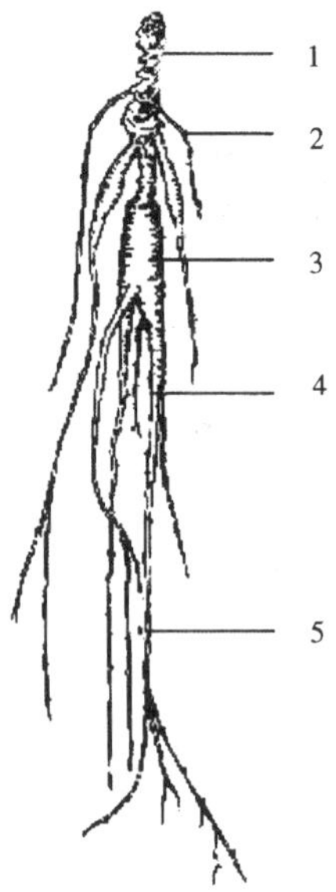

图 21-1 示人参药材

1. 茎痕（芦碗） 2. 不定根（艼） 3. 主根 4. 支根 5. 须根（珍珠疙瘩）

1. 性状鉴别

(1) 生晒参：主根圆柱形或纺锤形，表面黄白色或淡黄白色，上部有断续粗横纹，全体具明显的纵皱纹，须根上有不明显的疣状突起（习称“珍珠疙瘩”）。根茎（习称“芦头”）较短细，具茎痕（习称“芦碗”）及不定根（习称“艼”）。主根质硬，断面淡黄白色，形成层环棕黄色，皮部有黄棕色点状树脂道及放射状裂隙。香气特异；味微苦、甘。

(2) 红参：主根圆柱形或纺锤形，表面棕红色，半透明，有时上部棕黄色；有纵沟、皱纹及细根痕；质硬脆，断面平坦，角质样，中心色较浅。

(3) 生晒山参：主根与根茎等长或稍短，表面灰黄色，有浅皱纹，上部有细密环纹。根茎具多数密集的芦碗和艼，须根具较多而明显的珍珠疙瘩。常以“芦长碗密枣核艼，紧皮细纹珍珠须”概括其性状特征。

(4) 西洋参：呈圆柱形或长纺锤形，表面浅黄褐色或黄白色，有密集的细横纹及不规则纵皱纹。中下部可见呈叉状分枝的侧根或侧根痕。质坚，折断面平坦，淡黄色或粉白色，形成层环棕黄色。

2. 显微鉴别

(1) 生晒参主根横切面：木栓层为数列细胞。栓内层窄。韧皮部外侧有裂隙，内侧薄壁细胞排列较紧密，有树脂道散在，内含黄色分泌物。形成层成环。木质部射线宽广，导管单个散在或数个相聚，断续排列成放射状，导管旁偶有非木化的纤维。薄壁细胞含草酸钙簇晶。

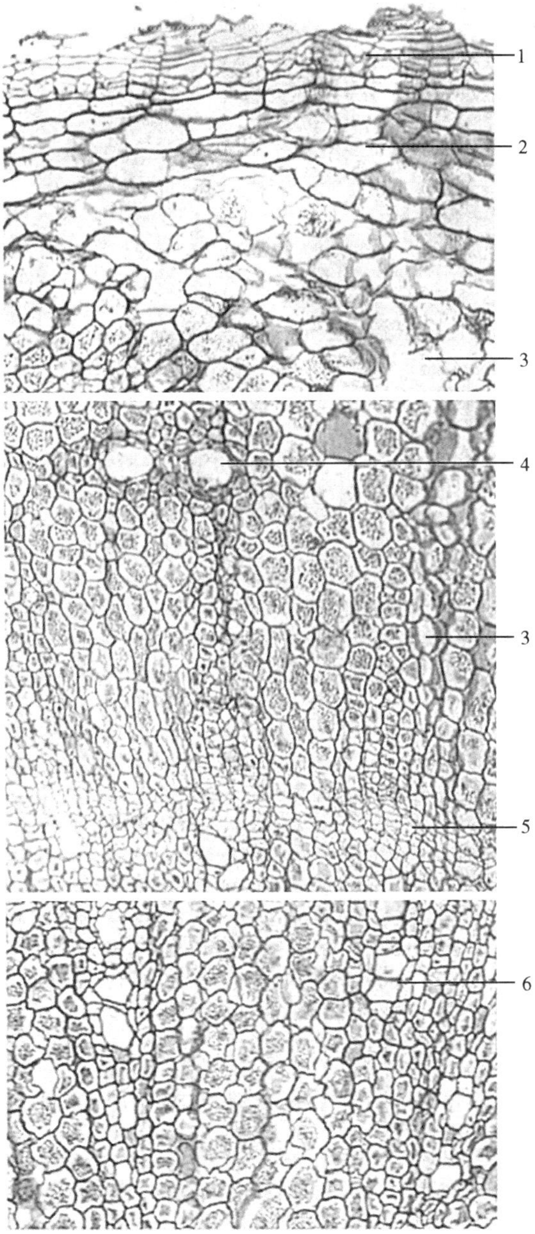

图 21－2　生晒参（根）横切面详图

1. 木栓层　2. 皮层　3. 韧皮部　4. 树脂道　5. 形成层　6. 木质部

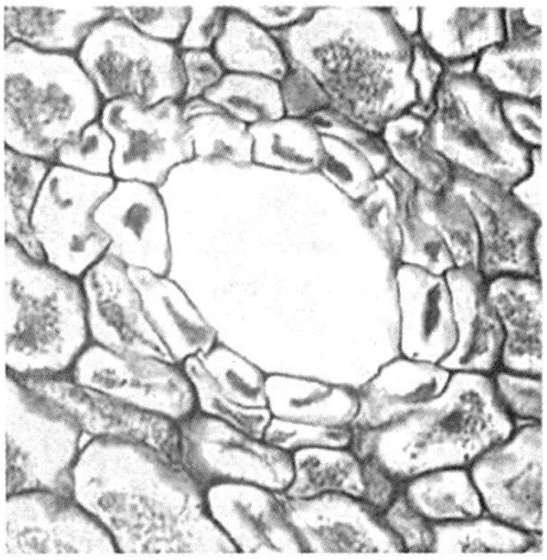

图 21－3　树脂道

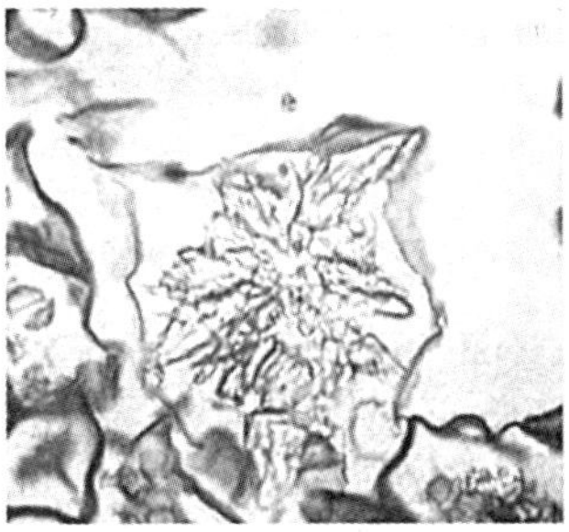

图 21－4　草酸钙簇晶

（2）生晒参粉末：①树脂道碎片易见，内含黄色块状分泌物。②草酸钙簇晶直径20～86 μm，多数棱角锐尖。③木栓细胞表面观呈类方形或多角形，垂周壁细波状弯曲。④导管主为网纹及梯纹导管。

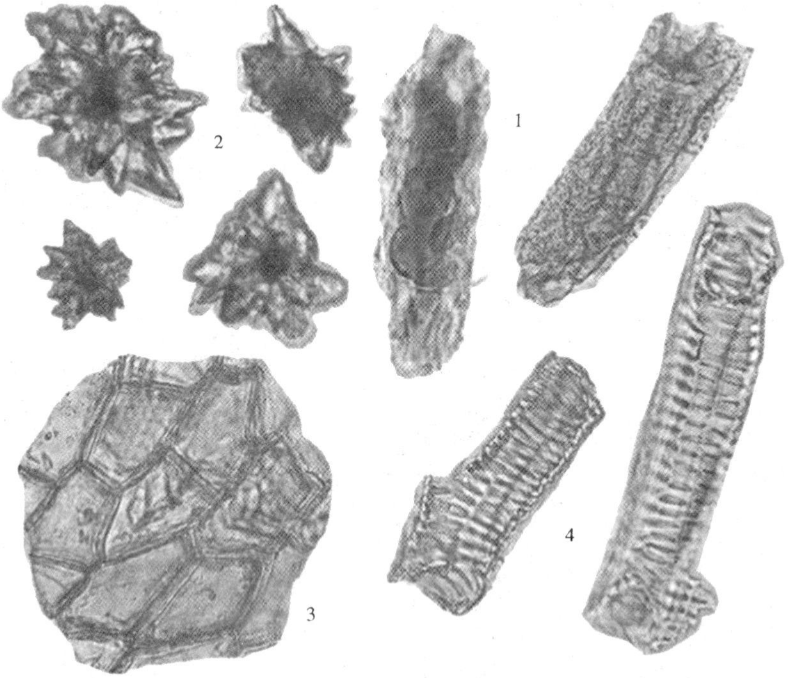

图 21－5　人参（根）粉末

1. 树脂道碎片　2. 草酸钙簇晶　3. 木栓细胞　4. 导管

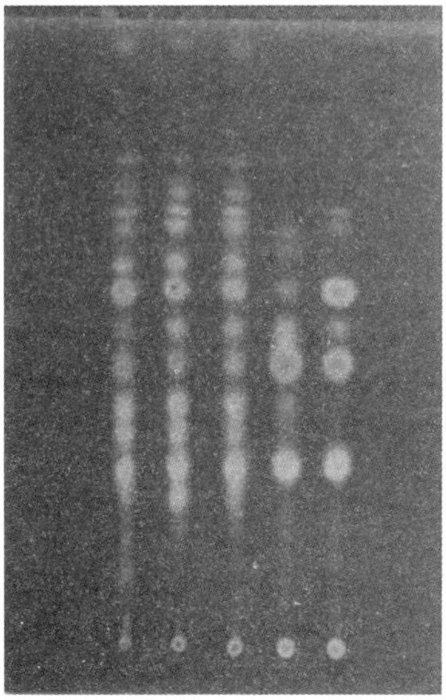

图 21－6　人参的薄层层析图谱

1. 生晒参　2. 红参　3. 朝鲜红参

4. 西洋参　5. 人参皂苷对照品

$S_1=Rb_1$，$S_2=Re$，$S_3=Rg_1$

3. 理化鉴别

(1) 取人参粉末 0.5 g，加 95% 乙醇 5 ml，振摇 5 分钟，滤过，取滤液少量，置蒸发皿中蒸干，滴加三氯化锑三氯甲烷饱和溶液，残渣显紫色。

(2) 取人参粉末 1 g，加三氯甲烷 40 ml，置水浴上回流 1 小时，弃去三氯甲烷液，药渣挥干残存溶剂，加水 0.5 ml 拌匀湿润后，加水饱和的正丁醇 10 ml，超声处理 30 分钟，吸取上清液，加氨试液 3 倍量，摇匀，放置分层，取上层液蒸干，残渣加 1 ml 甲醇溶解，作供试品溶液。再取人参皂苷 Rb_1、Re、Rg_1，加甲醇溶解，使成 2 mg/ml 的混合溶液，作对照品溶液。吸取上述两种溶液各 1～2 μl，分别点样于同一硅胶 G 薄层板（厚度 0.5 cm），以三氯甲烷－乙酸乙酯－甲醇－水 (15:40:22:10) 10℃以下放置后的下层溶液为展开剂，展开，取出，晾干，喷 10% 硫酸乙醇溶液，105℃ 加热至斑点显色清晰，置紫外光灯 (365 nm) 下观察，样品与对照品在相同位置显相同色斑。

4. DNA 分子遗传标记鉴定

用 RAPD、DNA 测序等方法鉴定人参属 3 种植物人参（*P. ginseng*）、西洋参（*P. quinquefolium*）和竹节参（*P. japonicus*）药材以及相关新鲜材料。采用 18SrRNA 基因片断通用引物对 18S F 和 18S R，通过 PCR 扩增，结果得到了约 1.8kb 片段的 PCR 产物。经过 DNA 测序发现 3 种药材间的 18SrRNA 基因片段上第 497、499、501 和 712 号核苷酸序列不同，可用来鉴别人参及其相关药材。进一步采用 *matK* 基因片断通用引物对 *matK* AF 和 *matK* 8R，经过 DNA 测序发现西洋参与人参、竹节参间的 *matK* 基因片段上核苷酸序列差异可用来鉴别人参与西洋参。

（1）18S rRNA 基因区 PCR 产物电泳图谱

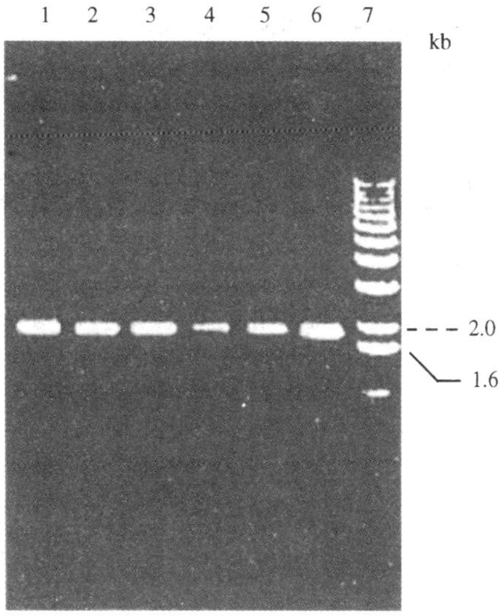

图 21－7　18S rRNA 基因区 PCR 产物电泳图谱
1. *P. ginseng*　2. *P. japonicus*　3. *P. quinquefolium*
4. Radix Ginseng　5. Radix Japonicus
6. Radix Quinquefolium　7. 1kb ladder

（2）DNA 测序

```
P. ginseng        481: ATAACAATAC CGGGCTGATT CAGTCTGGTA ATTGGAATGA 520
P. japonicus           ********** ******C*T* G********* **********
P. quinquefolium       ********** ******C*G* G********* **********
P. ginseng        681: CGATCGTCTC GTCCCTTCTG CCGGCGATGC GCTCCTGTCC 720
P. japonicus           ********** ********** ********** *T********
P. quinquefolium       ********** ********** ********** *C********
```

图 21－8　不同人参样品的 18S rRNA 基因序列（显示 497、499、501 和 712 号核苷酸碱基的不同）

5. 常见人参伪品的鉴别

（1）商陆：为商陆科植物商陆 *Phytolacca acinosa* Roxb. 或美洲商陆 *P. americana* L. 的根。表面红棕色或棕褐色。无芦头而有茎的残基。商陆根横切面木栓层多已除去，有同心性排列的三生维管束。有的薄壁细胞含草酸钙针晶。无草酸钙簇晶及树脂道。

（2）华山参根：为茄科植物华山参 *Physochlaina infundibularis* Kuang 的根。有短根茎，但无芦碗。表面黄棕色，具点状须根痕。华山参根横切面，残存的木栓层含棕色物。次生皮层及韧皮薄壁细胞含草酸钙砂晶。无树脂道与草酸钙簇晶，具生物碱反应，有毒。

（3）野豇豆根：为豆科植物野豇豆 *Vigna vexillata*（L.）Benth. 的根。野豇豆根表面灰棕色，有显著纵纹，无横纹，有豆腥气。木栓层多已除去。皮部、木部均含有纤维，不含草酸钙簇晶。

（4）土人参根：为马齿苋科植物锥花土人参 *Talinum paniculatum*（Jocq.）Gaertn. 的根。土人参根端有残茎而无芦头、芦碗，质坚实，断面平坦，中央常有大空腔，有的薄壁细胞含草酸钙簇晶，但无树脂道。

【实验作业】

1. 绘人参根横切面组织简图。
2. 绘人参粉末的草酸钙簇晶、树脂道碎片图。
3. 绘人参薄层色谱图。

【思考题】

1. 什么规格的人参中的人参皂苷含量最高？为什么？
2. 如何运用现代生物技术鉴别人参类药材？

21 Identification of Radix et Rhizoma Ginseng (Araliaceae)

Objectives

1. Master the description and microscopic identification of Radix et Rhizoma Ginseng.

2. Master the chemical constituents and physico-chemical identification on Radix et Rhizoma Ginseng.

3. Study the application of molecular tag technology on Radix et Rhizoma Ginseng.

4. Study the distinguishing characters of *Panax ginseng* and *P. quinquefolium*.

5. Study the distinguishing characters of *P. ginseng* and its adulterants.

Experiment Material

Crude drug specimens of *Panax ginseng* (Sun-dried Ginseng, Red ginseng) and *P. quinquefolium*; permanent mounts of Radix et Rhizoma Ginseng and powered Radix et Rhizoma Ginseng.

Experiment Methods

1. Description

Sun-dried Ginseng: Main roots fusiform or cylindrical, externally greyish-yellow; upper part or entire root exhibiting sparse, shallow, interrupted rootletsand coarse transverse striations and distinct longitudinal wrinkles; numerous slender rootlets with inconspicuous minute tubercles (Zhenzhugeda). Rhizomes (Lutou) mostly constricted and curved, bearing adven titious roots (Ding) and sparse depressed circular stem scars (Luwan). Texture relatively hard, fracture yellowish-white, cambium ring brownish-yellow, bark exhibiting yellow-brown dotted resin canals and radial clefts. Odour, characteristic; taste, slightly bitter and sweet.

Red ginseng: Main roots fusiform or cylindrical. Externally reddish-brown with translucent, occasionally exhibiting a few yellowish-brown; furrowed, longitudinal wrinkles and rootlet scars, the upper part exhibiting interrupted indistinct annulations. Texture hard and fragile, fracture even, horny.

Sun-dried Wild Ginseng: Main roots as long as or shorter than rhizome, externally greyish-yellow, longitudinally wrinkled, upper end with dense deep depressed annulations. Rhizome with numerous dense stem scars (Luwan) and adven titious roots (Ding), rootlets orderly arranged and showing some distinct warts, known as "pearl-like knot" (Zhenzhugeda).

American Ginseng: Fusiform, cylindrical or conical. Externally pale yellowish-brown or yellowish-white, exhibiting dense transverse striations and irregular longitudinal-wrinkles, and rootlet scars. The middle and lower part of the main root with 1 to several lateral roots or lateral roots scars. Texture heavy and hard, fracture even, yellowish-white, cambium ring brownish-yellow.

2. Microscopic identification

Transverse section:

Cork consisting of several rows of cells. Phelloderm narrow. Phloem showing clefts in the outer part, parenchymatous cells densely arranged and scattered with resin canals containing yellow secretions in the inner part. Cambium in a ring. Xylem rays broad, vessels singly scattered or grouped, interruptedly arranged radially, occasionally accompanied by non-lignified fibres. Parenchymatous cells containing clusters of calcium oxalate.

Powder:

(1) Fragments of resin canals containing yellow masses of secretion.

(2) Clusters of calcium oxalate 20～86 μm in diameter, with acute angles.

(3) Cork cells subsquare or polygonal, with thin and sinuous walls.

(4) Reticulate and scalariform vessels.

3. Physico-chemical identification

(1) To 0.5 g of the powder add 5 ml of ethanol. Shake for 5 minutes filter. Evaporate a small quantity of the filtrate to dryness in an evaporating dish. Add 3 drops of a saturated solution of antimony trichloride in chloroform, a violet colour is produced.

(2) To 1 g of the powder add 40 ml of chloroform, heat under reflux on a water bath for 1 hour, discard the chloroform layer, evaporate the residue to dryness. Moisten the residue with 0.5 ml of water. add 10 ml of *n*-buthanol saturated with water, ultrasonic treatment for 30 minutes. To the supernatant liquid add 3 volumes of ammonia TS, mix well, allow to stand, evaporate the supernatant liquid to dryness, dissolve the residue in 1 ml of methanol as the test solution. Dissolve ginsenosides Rb_1, Re, Rg_1 in methanol to produce a solution containing each of 2 mg per ml as the reference solution. Carry out the method for thin layer chromatography, using silica gel G as the coating substance (500 μm thick) and chloroform-ethyl acetate-methanol-water (15∶40∶22∶10) as the mobile phase. Apply separately to the plate 1～2 μl of

each of the two solutions. After developing and removal of the plate, dry it in air, spray with 10% solution of sulfuric acid in ethanol, heat at 105℃ for several minutes. Examine under sun-light and ultraviolet light (365 nm). The spots or fluorescent spots in the chromatogram obtained with the test solution correspond in position and colour to the spots in the chromatogram obtained with the reference drug solution. The three purplish-red spots in the chromatogram obtained with the test solution under sun-light correspond in position and color to the spots in the chromatogram obtained with the reference solution. A yellow and two orange fluorescent spots in the chromatogram obtained with the test solution under ultra-violet light (365 nm) correspond in position and color to the spots in the chromatogram obtained with the reference solution.

4. Identification with DNA genetic tag technology

To identify *Panax ginseng*, *P. quinquefolium*, *P. japonicus* and the relative fresh materials with the method of measuring the RAPD and DNA sequence. Adopting the general primers of 18SrRNA gene fragment, through PCR amplification of 18S F and 18S R results in about 1.8 kb PCR product. The difference of the 497th, 499th, 501th and 712th of nucleotide sequence among the 18SrRNA gene fragment of the 3 kinds of drugs, was found by measuring the DNA sequence, which can be used to identify *Panax ginseng* and the relative drugs. Further adopting the general primers of *matK* gene fragment, through measuring DNA sequence, the distinct nucleotide sequence of *matK* gene fragment among *P. quinquefolium*, *P. japonicus* and *P. ginseng*, can be used to identify *P. quinquefolium* and *P. ginseng*.

5. Identification of Radix Ginseng' adulterants

(1) Radix Phytolaccae: Radix Phytolaccae is the dried root of *Phytolacca acinosa* Roxb or *P. americana* L. Externally reddish brown or dark brown. Without rhizomes (Lutou) but bearing remains of stems. Transverse section of root, most cork removed. Fibro-vascular tissue forming tertiary structure, with several concentric cambium rings. Parenchymatous cells containing raphides of calcium oxalate, not containing clusters of calcium oxalate and resin canals.

(2) Radix Physochlainae: Radix Physochlainae is the dried root *of Physochlaina infundibularis* Kuang, family Solanaceae. Bearing short rhizoma without stem stars (Luwan), Externally yellowish brown, some rootlet scars appearing on the upper part. Transverse section of root with remains of cork containing brown substances. Secondary cortex and phloem parenchymatous cells containing sandy crystals of calcium oxalate, not containing clusters of calcium oxalate and resin canals. Alkaloid reaction is positive. Poisonous.

(3) Radix Vignae vexillatae: Radix Vignae vexillatae is the dried root of *Vigna vexillata* (L.) Benth, Family Leguminosae. Externally grayish brown with distinct

longitudinal wrinkles without transversal wrinkles. Odour, bean-like. Most cork removed. Both bark and wood containing fibers, not containing clusters of calcium oxalate.

(4) Radix Talini paniculati: Radix Talini paniculati is the dried root of *Talinum paniculatum* (Jocq.) Gaertn, Family Portulacaceae. The upper part bearing the remains of stem, without rhizomes (Lutou), depressed circular stem scars (Luwan), texture hard, fracture fairly even, the center usually hollowed. Parenchymatous cells sometimes containing clusters of calcium oxalate, not containing resin canals.

Laboratory Assignments

1. Make a diagram of the transverse section of Radix et Rhizoma Ginseng.

2. Make a drawing of the powdered Radix et Rhizoma Ginseng, and signify clusters of calcium oxalate and resin canals.

3. Make a drawing of TLC on Radix et Rhizoma Ginseng.

Questions

1. What specification of Radix et Rhizoma Ginseng contains the highest content of ginsenosides, and why ?

2. How to identify Radix et Rhizoma Ginseng with the modern biotechnology ?

实验二十二　伞形科生药——当归的鉴定

【实验目的】

1. 掌握当归性状、显微的主要鉴别特征。
2. 掌握当归的化学成分及理化鉴别方法。

【实验材料】

当归 *Angelica sinensis*（Oliv.）Diels 的生药标本；当归组织切片和当归药材粉末。

【实验方法】

1. 性状鉴别

根头（归头）及主根（归身）粗短，略成圆柱形，支根（归尾）2～10 多条，扭曲。表面黄棕色至棕褐色，有纵皱纹及横向皮孔，根头上端圆钝，残留多层鳞片状叶鞘残基。支根上粗下细，多扭曲，有少数须根痕。质较柔软，断面黄白色或淡黄棕色，皮部有多数棕色油点，形成层环黄棕色。有浓郁的香气，味甘、辛、微苦。

2. 显微鉴别

(1) 根横切面：木栓层为数列木栓细胞。皮层窄，有少数油室。韧皮部宽广，多裂隙，油室或油管类圆形，直径 60～220 μm，外侧较大，向内渐小，周围分泌细胞 6～10 个。形成层成环。木质部射线宽 3～10 列细胞，导管作放射状排列。

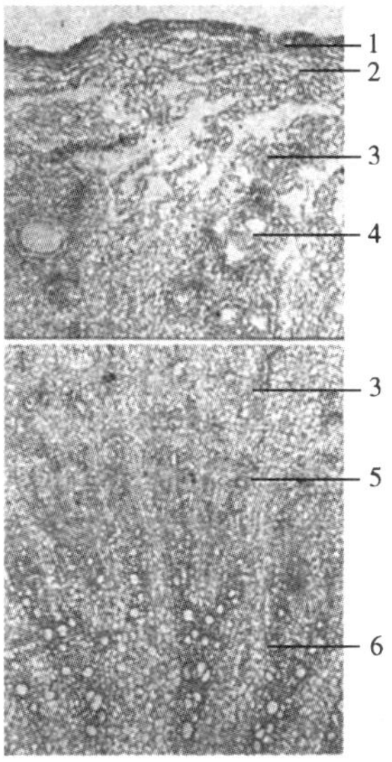

图 22-1　当归（根）横切面
1. 木栓层　2. 皮层　3. 韧皮部
4. 油室　5. 形成层　6. 木质部

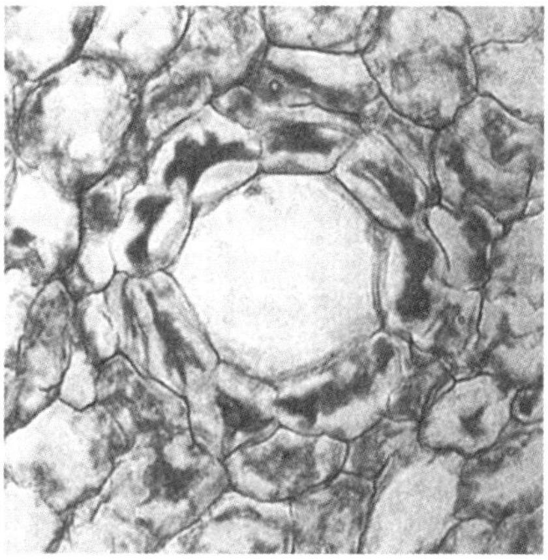

图 22-2　油室

（2）粉末淡黄棕色。

①韧皮薄壁细胞纺锤形，壁稍厚，表面有微细斜向交错的纹理，有时可见菲薄的横隔。

②梯纹及网纹导管多见，直径约至 80 μm。

③油室及油管碎片有时可见。

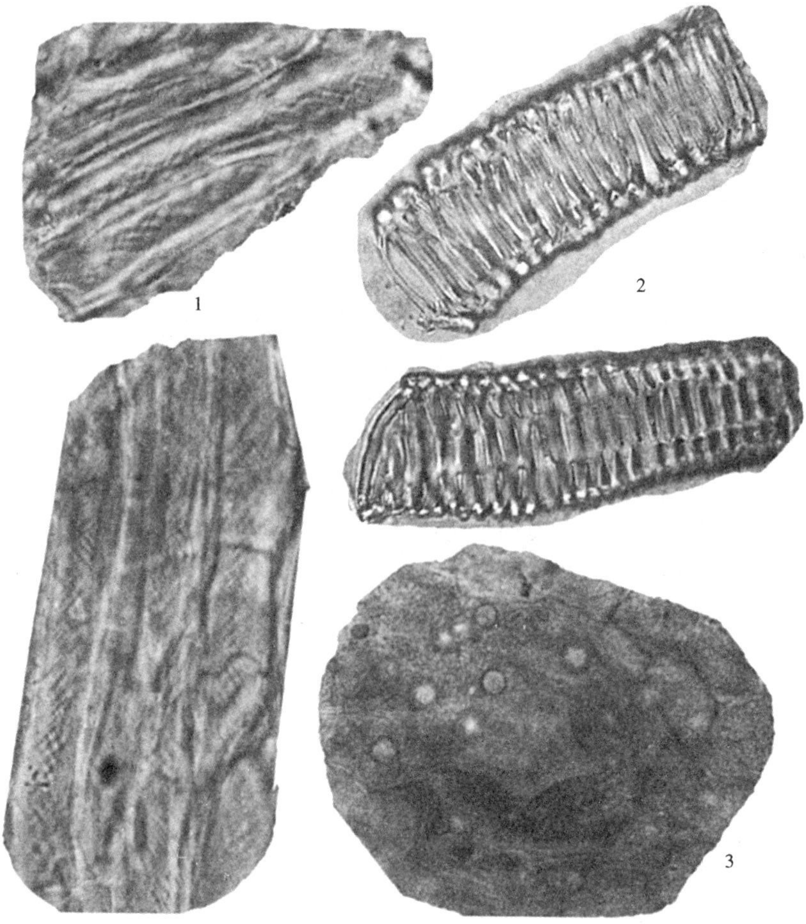

图 22－3　当归（根）粉末

1. 韧皮薄壁细胞　2. 梯纹及网纹导管　3. 油室

【实验作业】

1. 记述当归组织特征，绘横切面组织简图。

2. 记述当归粉末特征，绘韧皮薄壁细胞图。

【思考题】

1. 归头、归身、归尾各属当归哪个部位？各在功效上有何区别？以何地产者为道地药材？

2. 当归主含何种化学成分？

22 Identification of Radix Angelicae Sinensis (Umbelliferae)

Objectives

1. Master the description and microscopic identification of Radix Angelicae Sinensis.

2. Master the chemical constituents and physico-chemical identification on Radix Angelicae Sinensis.

Experiment Material

Crude drug specimens of *Angelicae sinensis* (Oliv.) Diels; permanent mounts of Radix Angelicae sinensis; powdered Radix Angelicae sinensis.

Experiment Methods

1. Description

Somewhat cylindrical, the root stock known as "Guitou", main root known as "Guishen", the branching root 2～10, twist, called "Guiwei ". Externally yellowish-brown to dark brown, longitudinally wrinkled and transversely lenticellate; the upper portion swollen, blunt and rounded, showing remains of stem and leaf sheaths; branching root, thick in the upper portion and thin in the lower portion, mostly twisted and exhibiting a few rootlet scars. Texture flexible, fracture yellowish-white or yellowish-brown, bark thick, showing brown oil spots, cambium ring yellowish-brown. Odour, strongly aromatic; taste, sweet, pungent and slightly bitter.

2. Microscopic identification

Transverse section of main root: Cork cells in several layers. Cortex narrow, scattered with a few oil cavities. Phloem broad, more cleft, oil cavities or oil tubes subround, 60～220 μm in diameter, relatively large on the outer side, gradually becoming small in wards, surrounded by 6～10 secretory cells. Cambium in a ring. Xylem rays 3～10 rows of cells wide; vessels arranged radiatively.

Powder: Pale yellowish-brown, Parenchymatous cells in phloem fusiform, walls slightly thickened, with very fine oblique crisscross striations, sometimes thin transverse septa visible. Scalariform and reticulate vessels frequent, up to 80 μm in diameter. Sometimes fragments of oil cavities visible.

Laboratory Assignments

1. Record the characters of transverse section of Radix Angelicae Sinensis, and make a diagram of transverse section of Radix Angelicae Sinensis.

2. Record the characters of powder of Radix Angelicae Sinensis, and make a drawing of parenchymatous cells in phloem.

Questions

1. Which parts of "Guitou", "Guishen" and "Guiwei" belong to respectively? What are the differences among the three on effect? where is the genuine crude drug from?

2. What constituents are mainly contained in Radix Angelicae Sinensis?

实验二十三　伞形科生药——小茴香的鉴定

【实验目的】

1. 掌握小茴香性状、显微的主要鉴别特征。
2. 掌握小茴香的化学成分及理化鉴别方法。
3. 熟悉小茴香中挥发油含量测定方法。

【实验材料】

小茴香 *Foeniculum vulgare* Mill. 的生药标本；小茴香果实组织切片；小茴香药材粉末。

【实验方法】

1. 性状鉴别

本品为双悬果，呈细椭圆形，有的稍弯曲，长 3～8 mm，直径 1.5～3 mm；表面黄绿色或淡黄棕色，两端略尖，顶端残留黄棕色突起的柱基，基部有细果柄；悬果瓣（分果）呈长椭圆形，背面有纵棱 5 条，接合面平坦；横切面略呈五边形，背面的四边约等长；香气特异，味微甜、辛。

2. 显微鉴别

分果横切面：外果皮为 1 列扁平细胞，外被角质层。中果皮纵棱处有维管束，其周围有多数木化网纹细胞；背面纵棱间各有大的椭圆形棕色油管 1 个，接合面有油管 2 个，共 6 个。内果皮为 1 列扁平薄壁细胞，细胞长短不一。种皮细胞扁长，含棕色物。胚乳细胞多角形，含多数糊粉粒，每个糊粉粒中含有细小草酸钙簇晶。

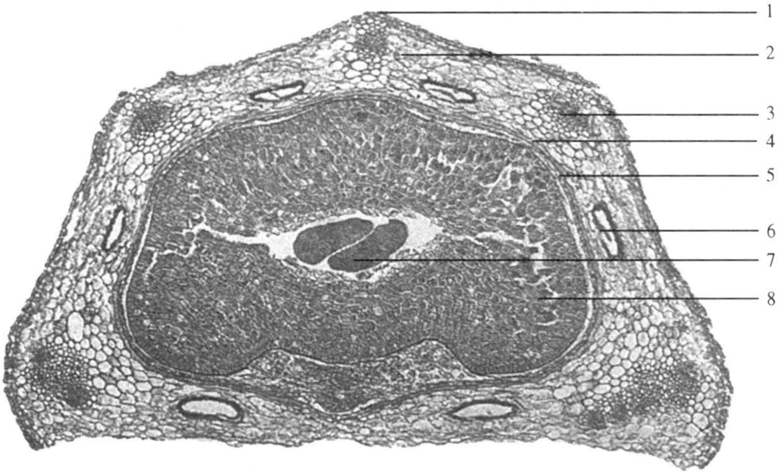

图 23－1　小茴香（果实）横切面

1. 外果皮　2. 中果皮　3. 维管束　4. 内果皮　5. 种皮　6. 油管　7. 胚　8. 胚乳

3. 理化鉴别

（1）取本品粉末0.5 g，加入乙醚适量，冷浸1小时，滤过，滤液浓缩至约1 ml，加0.4% 2,4 －二硝基苯肼2 mol/L盐酸溶液2～3滴，溶液显橘红色。（检查茴香脑）

（2）取本品粉末0.5 g，加乙醚适量，冷浸1小时，滤过，滤液浓缩至约1 ml，加7%盐酸羟胺甲醇液2～3滴，加20%氢氧化钾乙醇液3滴，在水浴上微热，冷却后，加稀盐酸调节pH至3～4，再加1%三氯化铁乙醇溶液1～2滴呈紫色（检查香豆素）。

（3）薄层层析：取本品粉末2 g，加乙醚20 ml，超声处理10分钟，滤过。将滤液浓缩至干，残渣用三氯甲烷溶解至1 ml，作供试品溶液。另取茴香醛对照品，加乙醇制成每1 ml含1 μl的溶液，作对照品溶液。吸取供试品溶液5 μl、对照品溶液1 μl，分别点样于同一硅胶G薄层板上，以石油醚（60～90℃）－乙酸乙酯（17:2.5）为展开剂，展距8 cm,取出，晾干后喷2,4 －二硝基苯肼试液。供试品色谱在与对照品色谱相应的位置上，显相同的橙红色斑点。

（4）挥发油含量测定：照挥发油测定法测定。本品含挥发油不得少于1.5%（ml/g）。

【实验作业】

1. 绘小茴香分果的横切面组织简图。
2. 记述小茴香理化鉴别步骤与结果。
3. 记录挥发油的读数，样品中挥发油的含量是否符合《中国药典》规定？

【思考题】

什么是镶嵌细胞？

23 Identification of Fructus Foeniculi (Umbelliferae)

Objectives

1. Master the description and microscopic identification of Fructus Foeniculi.

2. Master the chemical constituents and physico-chemical identification on Fructus Foeniculi.

3. Familiar with the method for determination of volatile oil from Fructus Foeniculi.

Experiment Material

Crude drug specimens of *Foeniculum vulgare* Mill.; permanent mounts of Fructus Foeniculi and powdered Fructus Foeniculi.

Experiment Methods

1. Description

Cremocarp, elliptical, some slightly curved, 3～8 mm long, 1.5～3 mm in diameter. Externally yellowish-green or pale yellow, tapering slightly towards both ends, apex bearing remains of yellowish-brown projecting stylopodium, having a small fruit stalk at the base. Mericarp elongated-elliptical, with each dorsal surface bearing five ribs and commissural surface flattened and broad. Transverse section showing a pentagonal, the four sides of dorsal surface nearly equal in length. Odour, characteristically aromatic; taste, slightly sweet and pungent.

2. Microscopic identification

Transverse section of mericarp: Exocarp consisting of 1 layer of flattened cells, covered cuticle at outside. Mesocarp with 5 ribs each containing a vascular bundle surrounded by numerous lignified reticulate cells. Vittae 6, large, elliptical and brown, 4 of them situated in the dorsal between every 2 ribs and 2 in the commissural. Endocarp consisting of 1 layer of flattened thin-walled cells varying in length. The testa cells compressed and elongated, containing brown contents. Endosperm cells polygonal, filled with aleurone grains, each embedding a minute cluster of calcium oxalate.

3. Physico-chemical identification

(1) To 0.5 g of the powder add moderation of ether, macerate for 1 hour, filter. Evaporate the filtrate to 1 ml, add 2～3 drops of a 0.4% solution of 2,4 - dinitro-

phenylhydrazine in 2 mol/L hydrochloric acid, orange-red is produced. (Examine anethole)

(2) To 0.5 g of the powder add moderation of ether, macerate for 1 hour and filter. Evaporate the filtrate to 1 ml, add 2~3 drops of 7% solution of hydroxylamine hydrochloride in methanol, add 3 drops of 20% solution of potassium hydroxide in methanol, slightly heat under reflux on a water bath, cool, add dilute hydrochloric acid to adjust pH to 3~4, then add 1~2 drops of 1% solution of ferric chloride in ethanol, purple is produced.

(3) To 2 g of the powder add 20 ml of ether, ultrasonic treatment for 10 minutes, filter and evaporate the filtrate to dryness. Dissolve the residue in 1 ml of chloroform as the test solution. Dissolve anisaldehyde CRS in ethanol to produce a solution containing 1 μg per ml as the reference solution. Using silica gel G as the coating substance and a mixture of petroleum ether (60~90℃) -ethyl acetate (17:2.5) as the mobile phase. Apply 5 μl of test solution and 1 μl of reference solution to the plate. After developing 8 cm and removal of the plate, dry it in air. Spray with a solution of dinitrophenylhydrazine TS. The orange-red spot in the chromatogram obtained with the test solution corresponds in position and colour to the spot in the chromatogram obtained with the reference solution.

(4) Carry out the method for determination of volatile oil. It contains not less than 1.5% (ml/g) of volatile oil.

Laboratory Assignments

1. Make a diagram of the transverse section of mericarp of Fructus Foeniculi.
2. Record the procedure and result of identification on Fructus Foeniculi.
3. Note reading of volatile oil, and whether the content of volatile oil in sample was up to rules of the Chinese pharmacopoeia?

Questions

What is incrusted cell?

实验二十四　马钱科生药——马钱子的鉴定

【实验目的】

1. 掌握马钱子性状、显微的主要鉴别特征。
2. 了解马钱子的化学成分及理化鉴别方法。

【实验材料】

马钱 *Strychnos nux-vomica* L. 的生药标本；马钱子组织切片及马钱子粉末。

【实验方法】

1. 性状鉴别

本品呈扁圆纽扣状，常一面隆起，一面稍凹下，直径 1.2～3 cm，厚 0.3～0.6 cm。表面密被灰棕色或灰绿色茸毛，自中间向四周呈辐射状排列，有丝样光泽。边缘稍隆起，较厚，有突起的珠孔，底面中心有突起的圆点状种脐。质坚硬，平行剖面可见淡黄白色胚乳，角质状，子叶心形，叶脉 5～7 条。无臭，味极苦。

2. 显微鉴别

组织横切面：种皮表皮细胞分化成单细胞毛，向一方斜伸，长 500～1100 μm，宽 25 μm以上；基部膨大，石细胞状，直径约 75 μm，壁极厚，强木化，有纵长扭曲的纹孔；毛的体部约有 10 条肋状木化增厚条纹。种皮内层为颓废的棕色薄壁细胞。内胚乳细胞壁厚约 25 μm，隐约可见胞间连丝，细胞内含脂肪油滴和糊粉粒。

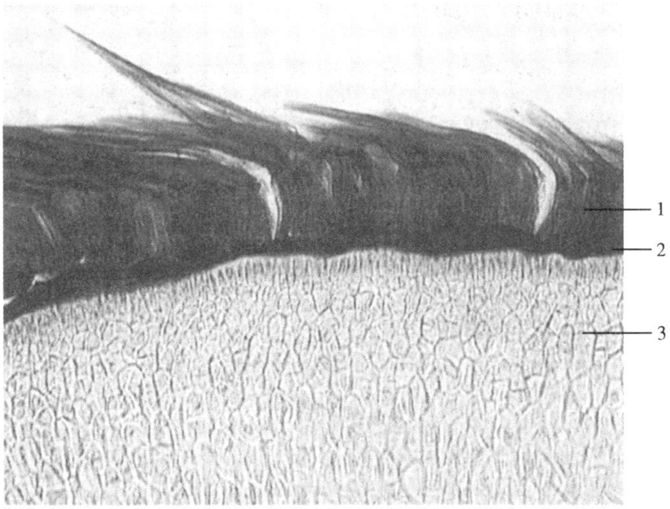

图 24－1　马钱子横切面

1. 种皮　2. 种皮表皮细胞　3. 内胚乳

3. 理化鉴别

（1）取本品干燥种子的胚乳作切片，加 1% 钒酸铵的硫酸溶液 1 滴，胚乳即显紫色；另取胚乳切片，加发烟硝酸 1 滴，即显橙红色。

（2）取本品粉末 0.5 g，加三氯甲烷－乙醇（10∶1）混合液 5 ml 与浓氨试液 0.5 ml，密塞，振摇 5 分钟，放置 2 小时，滤过，滤液作供试品溶液。另取士的宁和马钱子碱对照品，加三氯甲烷制成每毫升各含 2 mg 的混合溶液，作对照品溶液。吸取上述两种溶液各 10 μl，分别点于同一硅胶 G 薄层板上，以甲苯－丙酮－乙醇－浓氨试液（4∶5∶0.6∶0.4）为展开剂，展开，取出，晾干，喷稀碘化铋钾试液。供试品色谱中，在与对照品色谱相应位置上，显相同颜色（橙色）的斑点。

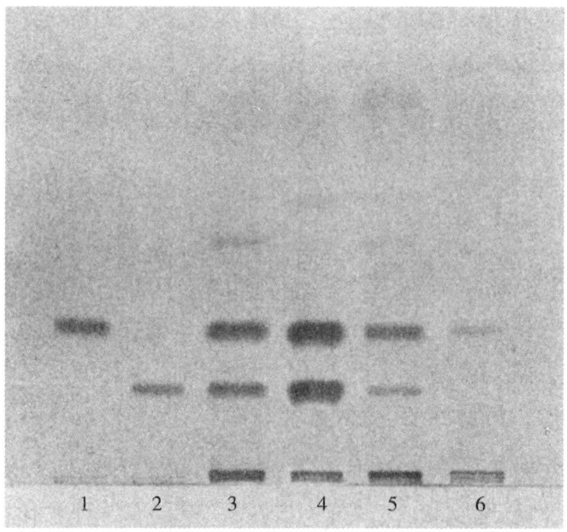

图 24－2　马钱子薄层层析图谱

1. 番木鳖碱　2. 马钱子碱　3. 马钱子（对照药材）

4. 云南马钱（对照药材）　5. 马钱子（商品）　6. 制马钱

【实验作业】

1. 绘马钱子横切面显微特征图，示种皮表皮非腺毛。
2. 记录马钱子理化鉴别结果。

【思考题】

1. 马钱子的毒性成分与有效成分是什么？
2. 马钱子的炮制目的是什么？

24 Identification of Semen Strychni (Loganiaceae)

Objectives

1. Master the description and microscopic identification of Semen Strychni.

2. Study the chemical constituents and physico-chemical identification on Semen Strychni.

Experiment Material

Crude drug specimens of *Strychnos nux-vomica* L.; Permanent mounts of semen of *Strychnos nux-vomica*; powdered Semen Strychni.

Experiment Methods

1. Description

Button-shaped, frequently one side prominent and the other slightly dented, 1.2～3 cm in diameter, 0.3～0.6 cm thick. Outer surface closely covered with greyish-brown or greyish-green silky hairs, radiating from center to circumference, silky-lustrous. Edge slightly prominent, relatively thick, with a protuberant micropyle; a prominent dot-like hilum in center of the bottom surface. Texture hard, pale yellowish-white, endosperm visible in horizontal section, horny, cotyledons cordate, with 5～7 veins. Odourless; taste, extremely bitter.

2. Microscopic identification

Transverse section: The inner wall of epidermal cells of testa differentiated to singular cell hair, declining to one direction, 500～1100 μm long, above 25 μm wide; enlarged at base like a stone cell, 75 μm in diameter, great thickened-walls, strongly lignified, with lengthwise twisty pit; about 10 rib-likely lignified thickness on body of hair. Inner testa was obliterated brown parenchymatous cell. Thickened-walled cells of endosperm about 25 μm, sometimes plasmodesmata can be seen, containing fatty oil and aleurone grains.

3. Physico-chemical identification

(1) To a section of endosperm of the dried seed add 1 drop of a 1% solution of ammonium vanadate in sulfuric acid; a violet color is produced. To another section of endosperm add 1drop of fuming nitric acid; an orange-red color is produced.

(2) Extract 0.5 g of the powder with 5 ml of a mixture of chloroform-ethanol

(10∶1) and 0.5 ml of concentrated ammonia TS in a stopper conical flask by shaking for 5 minutes, allow to stand for 2 hours, filter and use the filtrate as the test solution. Dissolve strychnine CRS and brucine CRS in chloroform to produce a solution containing 2 mg of each per ml as the reference solution. Using silica gel G as the coating substance and toluene-acetone-ethanol-concentrate ammonia (4∶5∶0.6∶0.4) as the mobile phase. Apply separately 10 each of the two solutions to the plate. After developing and removal of the plate, dry it in air, spray with potassium iodobismuthate TS. The spots in the chromatogram obtained with the test solution correspond in position and color to the spots in the chromatogram obtained with the reference solution.

Laboratory Assignments

1. Make a diagram of the transverse section of Semen Strychni, and signify epidermal non-glandular hairs of testa.
2. Record the results of physico-chemical identification on Semen Strychni.

Questions

1. What are venomous constituents and effective constituents of Semen Strychni?
2. What is the purpose of processing Semen Strychni?

实验二十五　唇形科生药——薄荷的鉴定

【实验目的】

1. 掌握薄荷性状及显微的主要鉴别特征。
2. 熟悉薄荷的化学成分及理化鉴别方法。
3. 熟悉唇形科植物的主要性状与显微鉴别特征。
4. 熟悉全草类生药的鉴别要点。

【实验材料】

薄荷 *Mentha haplocalyx* Briq. 的生药标本；茎横切片、叶横切片及药材粉末。

【实验方法】

1. 性状鉴别

茎呈方柱形，有时对生分枝；表面黄棕色或带紫色，有明显的节，节间长 2～5 cm；棱角处有柔毛；质脆，断面白色，中空。叶卷曲皱缩，长椭圆形或卵形，有凹点状腺鳞。茎上部腋生轮伞花序，花冠多数存在，淡紫色。叶揉搓时有特异清凉的香气；味辛凉。

2. 显微鉴别

（1）茎横切面：呈四方形。表皮为 1 列长方形细胞。皮层薄壁细胞数列，排列疏松，四棱角处由厚角细胞组成。内皮层明显。韧皮部狭窄。形成层成环。木质部在四棱处发达。髓薄壁细胞大，中心常有空洞。

（2）叶横切面：上表皮细胞呈长方形,下表皮细胞细小扁平,有气孔;上下表皮有多数凹陷,内有大型特异的扁球形腺鳞。叶肉栅栏组织为 1～2 列细胞,海绵组织为 4～5 列细胞,叶肉细胞含针簇状橙皮苷结晶。主脉维管束外韧型,韧皮部和木质部外侧有厚角组织。

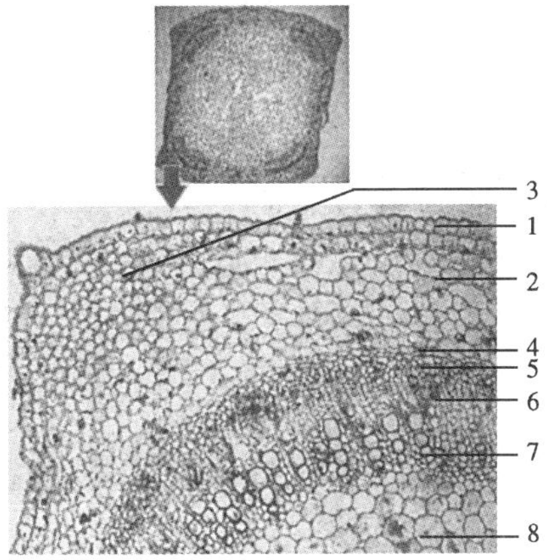

图 25－1　薄荷茎横切面详图

1. 表皮细胞　2. 皮层　3. 厚角细胞　4. 内皮层　5. 韧皮部　6. 形成层　7. 木质部　8. 髓部

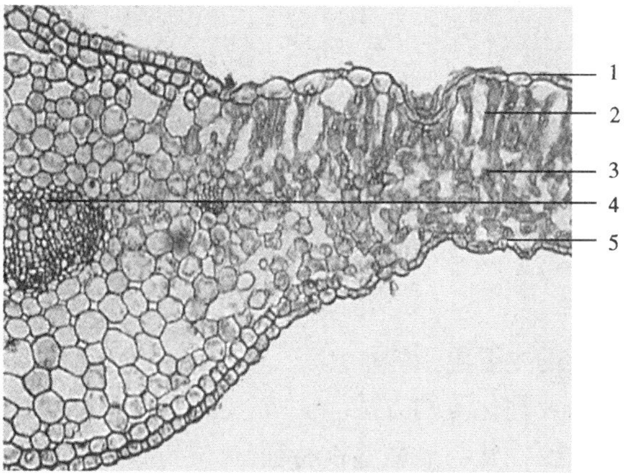

图 25－2　薄荷叶组织横切面

1. 表皮细胞　2. 栅栏组织　3. 海绵组织　4. 主脉维管束　5. 下表皮

（3）薄荷粉末：

①腺鳞头部顶面观呈类圆形，侧面观扁球形，6～8 细胞；柄单细胞。

②非腺毛完整者 1～8 细胞，稍弯曲，疣状突起较细密。

③叶片下表皮细胞壁弯曲，细胞中含橙皮苷结晶；气孔直轴式。

④橙皮苷结晶存在于茎、叶表皮细胞及薄壁细胞中，淡黄色，略成扇形或不规则形。

⑤茎表皮细胞表面观呈类长方形或类多角形，垂周壁稍厚，表面有角质纹理。

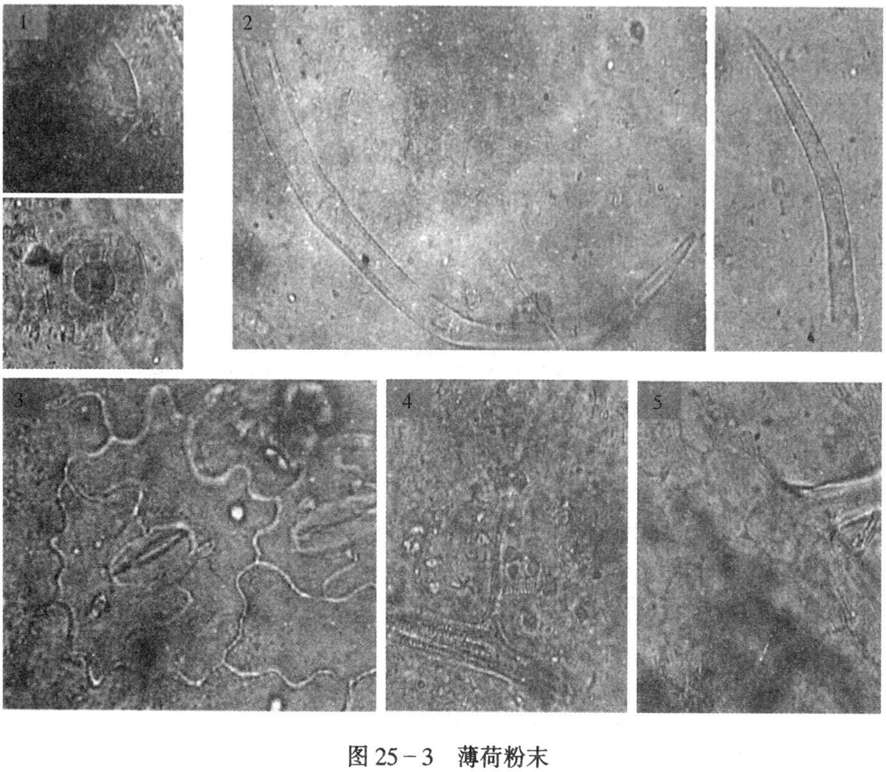

图 25－3　薄荷粉末

1. 腺鳞　2. 非腺毛　3. 叶片下表皮细胞　4. 橙皮苷结晶　5. 茎表皮细胞

3. 理化鉴别

（1）取本品叶的粉末少量，经微量升华得油状物，略放置，镜检，渐见有针簇状薄荷醇结晶析出；加浓硫酸 2 滴及香荚兰醛结晶少许，显橙黄色，再加蒸馏水 1 滴，变紫红色。

（2）薄层层析：取粉末 0.5 g，加石油醚（60～90℃）5 ml，冷浸半小时，滤过，滤液作供试品溶液。另取薄荷脑 2 mg 溶于 1 ml 三氯甲烷作对照品溶液。吸取上述供试品溶液、对照品溶液各 10 μl，分别点样于同一硅胶 G 薄层板，以苯:丙酮（9:1）为展开剂，展距 10 cm，取出，晾干，喷 5%香草醛硫酸试液，薄荷醇显玫瑰色，供试液在相同位置有相同色斑（加热或放置较长时间，色斑消失）。

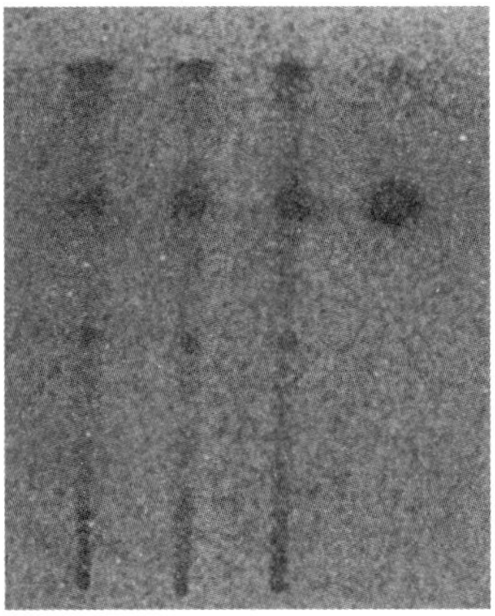

图 25－4　薄荷薄层层析图谱

1. 商品薄荷　2. 商品薄荷　3. 商品薄荷　4. 薄荷脑

【实验作业】

1. 绘薄荷茎横切面简图及叶粉末显微特征图，示腺鳞、非腺毛、表皮细胞及气孔。
2. 记录薄荷理化鉴别步骤及反应结果，说明其反应原理。

【思考题】

1. 唇形科全草类生药有哪些共同的性状与显微特征？
2. 双子叶植物草质茎的次生构造与木质茎的主要区别是什么？

25 Identification of Herba Menthae (Labiatae)

Objectives

1. Master the description and microscopic identification of Herba Menthae.

2. Familiar with the chemical constituents and the physico-chemical identification of Herba Menthae.

3. Familiar with the main description and microscopic identification of plants on Family Labiatae.

4. Familiar with the identification of Herbs.

Experiment Material

Crude drug specimens of *Mentha haplocalx*; permanent mounts of stem and leaf from *Mentha haplocalx*, powder of Herba Menthae.

Experiment Methods

1. Description

Stem square, sometimes with opposite branches; externally yellowish-brown or purplish-brown, with distinct nodes, internodes 2 ~ 5 cm long; the angular regions pubescent; texture fragile, fracture white, pith hollowed. Lamina crumpled and rolled, long-elliptical or ovate, bearing concave dotted grandular scales. Verticillaster axillary, coralla mostly existing, pale purple. Odour, characteristic and aromatic after rubbing leaves; taste, pungent and cool.

2. Microscopic identification

(1) Transverse section of stem: squre. Epidermal cells, rectangle, 1 layer. Parenchymatous cells, several layers, arranged laxly, four angular regions consisting of collenchyma cells. Endodermis pubescent. Phloem narrow. Cambium in ring. Xylem developed on the four angular regions. Parenchymatous cells of pith large, pith often hollowed.

(2) Transverse section of leaf: The upper epidermal cells, rectangle, the lower epidermal cells, small and flattened, with stomata; the upper and lower epidermis, numerous pitted, with large and characteristic flattened-spherical glandular scales. Palisade tissue consisting of 1 ~ 2 layers cells, spongy tissue 4 ~ 5 layers of cells, mesophyll tissue containing needle-cluster crystals of hesperidin. Vascular bundles of main vein collateral, collenchyma tissue on the out side of phloem and xylem.

(3) Powder of Herba Menthae

① The head of glandular scales, round in surface view; flattened-rounded in lateral view, 6~8 cells; an unicellular stalk.

② Non-glandular hairs, the whole 1~8 cells, slightly curved, warty close.

③ The lower epidermal cells of lamina, walls curved, containing crystals of hesperidin; stomata, diacytic.

④ Crystals of hesperidin occurring in epidermal and parenchymatous cells of stems and leaves, pale yellow, scallop or irregularly shaped.

⑤ The epidermal cells of stem in surface view rectangle-like or polygon-like, anticlinal walls slightly thick, cornification striation on the surface.

3. Physico-chemical identification

(1) Examine the oily matter obtained from the microsublimation of a small quantity of the leaf powder after standing for a little while, gradually educt needle-cluster crystals of menthol; add 2 drops of sulfuric acid and a small quantity of vanillin crystal, a orange-yellow colour is produced, turning to purplish-red on adding 1 drop of water.

(2) TLC: To 0.5 g of the powder add 5 ml of petroleum ether(60~90℃), allow to stand for 30 minutes, filter and use the filtrate as the test solution. Dissolve 2 mg of menthol CRS in 1 ml of chloroform to produce a solution as the reference solution. Using silica gel G as the coating substance and a mixture of benzene-acetone (9:1) as the mobile phase. Apply separately to the plate 10 μl of each of the solutions. After developing 10 cm and removal of the plate, dry it in air. Spray with a 0.5% mixture of vanillin in sulfuric acid, the spot of menthol is rosy, the spot in the chromatogram obtained with the test solution corresponds in position and colour to the spot in the chromatogram obtained with the reference solution (heating or standing for long, the spot disappears).

Laboratory Assignments

1. Make a drawing of the transverse section of stem from *Mentha haplocalyx* and the microscopic characteristic drawing of the powder from leaf, show the glandular scales, non-glandular hairs, epidermal cells and stomata.

2. Record the procedure and result of physico-chemical identification, explaining the reaction principles.

Questions

1. What are the mutual descriptions and microscopic characteristics of herbs from Family Labiatae?

2. What are the main differences of secondary structure between herbaceous stem and xylon stem of dicotyledon?

实验二十六　忍冬科生药——金银花的鉴定及质量标准的制定

【实验目的】

1. 掌握金银花性状、显微的主要鉴别特征。
2. 掌握金银花的化学成分及理化鉴别方法。
3. 了解金银花类生药的鉴别特征。

【实验材料】

忍冬(*Lonicera japonica* Thunb.)的生药标本,金银花药材粉末。

【实验方法】

1. 性状鉴别

金银花:呈细棒槌状,上粗下细,略弯曲,长 1.3～5.5 cm,上部直径约 3 mm,下部直径约 1.5 mm。表面黄白色或绿白色(贮久色渐深),密被短柔毛。偶见叶状苞片。花萼绿色,先端 5 裂,裂片有毛,长约 2 mm。开放时花冠筒状,先端二唇形;雄蕊 5 个,附于筒壁,黄色;雌蕊 1 个,子房无毛。气清香,味淡、微苦。

2. 显微鉴别

有两种类型的腺毛,一种腺毛头部倒圆锥形,顶部稍平坦,侧面观约 10～33 细胞,排成 2～4 层,直径 48～108 μm,柄 1～5 细胞, 长 70～700 μm;另一种头部呈类圆形或扁圆形,约 6～20 细胞,直径 24～80 μm,柄 2～4 细胞,长 24～80 μm。头部的分泌细胞含黄棕色分泌物。厚壁非腺毛多单细胞,表面有微细疣状突起,有的具角质螺纹;另有极多薄壁非腺毛,甚长,表面有微细疣状突起。花粉粒类球形,具 3 孔沟,表面有细密短刺及细颗粒状雕纹。

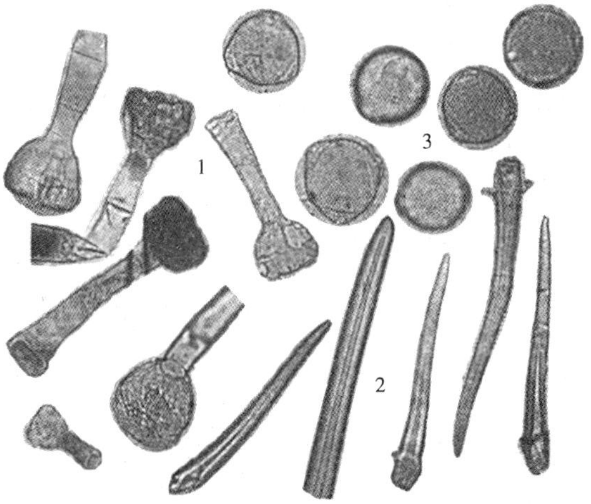

图 26－1　金银花粉末

1. 腺毛　2. 非腺毛　3. 花粉粒

3. 理化鉴别

取本品粉末 0.2 g，加甲醇 5 ml，放置 12 小时，滤过，滤液作供试品溶液。另取绿原酸对照品，加甲醇制成每 1 ml 含 1 mg 的溶液，作对照品溶液。吸取供试品溶液 10～20 μl、对照品溶液 10 μl 分别点于同一以羧甲基纤维素钠为黏合剂的硅胶 H 薄层板上，以醋酸丁酯－甲酸－水（7:2.5:2.5）的上层溶液为展开剂，展开，取出，晾干，置紫外灯（365 nm）下检视。供试品色谱中，在与对照品色谱相应的位置上，显相同颜色的荧光斑点。

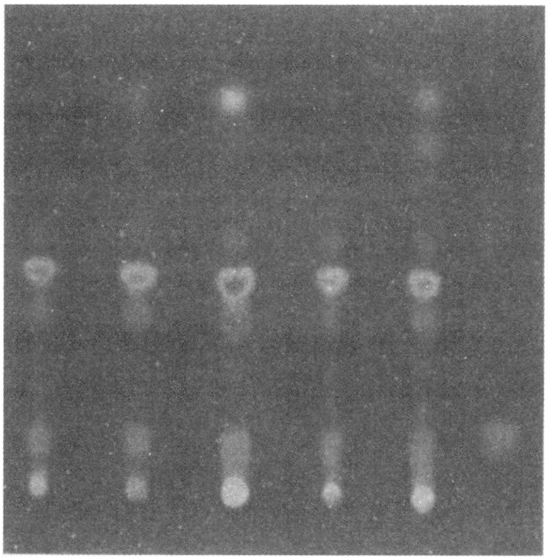

1　2　3　4　5　6

图 26－2　金银花薄层层析图谱

1. 金银花（河南密县）　2. 金银花（河南封丘）　3. 金银花（山东平邑）
4. 金银花（南京）　5. 金银花（商品）　6. 绿原酸（对照品）

4. 含量测定

（1）绿原酸　照《中国药典》2005 年版高效液相色谱法测定。

色谱条件与系统适用性试验　以十八烷基硅烷键合硅胶为填充剂；以乙腈－0.4% 磷酸溶液（13:87）为流动相；检测波长为 327 nm。理论板数按绿原酸峰计算应不低于 1000。

对照品溶液的制备　精密称取绿原酸对照品适量，置棕色量瓶中，加 50% 甲醇制成每 1 ml 含 40 μg 的溶液，即得（10℃以下保存）。

供试品溶液的制备　取本品粉末（过四号筛）约 0.5 g，精密称定，置具塞锥形瓶中，精密加入 50% 甲醇 50 ml，称定重量，超声处理（功率 250 W，频率 35 kHz）30 分钟，放冷，再称定重量，用 50% 甲醇补足减失的重量，摇匀，滤过，精密量取续滤液 5 ml，置 25 ml 棕色量瓶中，加 50% 甲醇至刻度，摇匀，即得。

测定法　分别精密吸取对照品溶液与供试品溶液各 5～10 μl，注入液相色谱仪，测定，即得。

本品按干燥品计算，含绿原酸（$C_{16}H_{18}O_9$）不得少于 1.5%。

（2）木犀草苷　照《中国药典》2005年版高效液相色谱法测定。

色谱条件与系统适用性试验　以十八烷基硅烷键合硅胶为填充剂；以乙腈为流动相A，以0.5%冰醋酸溶液为流动相B，按下表进行梯度洗脱；检测波长为350 nm。理论板数按木犀草苷峰计算应不低于2000。

时间（min）	流动相A（%）	流动相B（%）
0～30	10→30	90→70

对照品溶液的制备　精密称取木犀草苷对照品适量，加70%乙醇制成每1 ml含40 μg的溶液，即得。

供试品溶液的制备　取本品细粉（过四号筛）约3 g，精密称定，置具塞锥形瓶中，精密加入70%乙醇50 ml，称定重量，超声处理（功率250 W，频率35 kHz）1小时，放冷，再称定重量，用70%乙醇补足减失的重量，摇匀，滤过，取续滤液，即得。

测定法　分别精密吸取对照品溶液与供试品溶液各10 μl，注入液相色谱仪，测定，即得。

本品按干燥品计算，含木犀草苷（$C_{21}H_{20}O_{11}$）不得少于0.10%。

【实验作业】

1. 绘金银花粉末特征图，示腺毛、非腺毛及花粉粒。
2. 查阅文献资料，结合实验结果，起草金银花质量标准。

【思考题】

同属多种植物的花蕾作山银花入药，《中国药典》2005年版收载的有忍冬科植物红腺忍冬 *Lonicera hypoglauca* Miq.、山银花 *L. confusa* DC. 和灰毡毛忍冬 *L. macranthoides* Hand.-Mazz.，这3种植物的花蕾与忍冬的花蕾在性状和显微特征上有哪些异同？

26 Identification of Flos Lonicerae Japonicae (Caprifoliaceae) and the Stipulation of Drug Standards of Quality Control

Objectives

1. Master the description and microscopic identification of Flos Lonicerae Japonicae.

2. Master the properties of chemical constituents and physico-chemical identification on Flos Lonicerae Japonicae.

3. Study the distinguishing characters of crude drug of Flos Lonicerae.

Experiment Material

Crude drug specimens of Flos Lonicera Japonicae (*Lonicera japonica* Thunb), powder of Flos Lonicerae Japonicae.

Experiment Methods

1. Description

Flower of *Lonicera japonica*: Clavate, stout in upper part and tapered downwards, slightly curved, 1.3~5.5 cm long, about 3 mm in diameter in upper part and 1.5 mm in diameter in lower part. Externally yellowish-white or greenish-white, gradually darken on keeping, densely pubescent. Lobiform bracts occasionally visible. Calyx green, 5-lobed at the apex, lobes pubescent, about 2 mm long. Corolla tubular when open, apex 2-lipped; stamens 5, epipetalous, yellow; pistil 1, ovary glabrous. Odour, delicately aromatic; taste, weak and slightly bitter.

2. Microscopic identification

Powder: Two kinds of glandular hairs visible, one, the head obconical, somewhat flat at summit, composed of 10~33 cells which arranged in 2~4 layers, 48~108 μm in diameter, stalk of 1~5 cells, 70~700 μm long; the other, head subround or flattened-rounded, relatively small, consisting of 6~20 cells, 24~80 μm in diameter, stalk of 2~4 cells, 24~80 μm in length. Head cell of glandular hairs containing yellowish-brown masses of secretion. Non-glandular hairs unicellular, 2-typed, one, wall somewhat thick, having slightly warty protrudings and warts with uni-or bi-spiral; the other, wall thin, relatively long, having slightly warty protrudings. Pollens spheroical, out walls bearing meticulous close needlings and spine-like protrudings, apertures 3.

3. Physico-chemical identification

To 0.2 g of the powder add 5 ml of methanol, macerate for 12 hours, filter, the filtrate is used as test solution. Dissolve chlorogenic acid CRS in methanol to produce a solution containing 1 mg per ml as the reference solution. Carry out the method for thin layer chromatogrphy, using silica gel H containing sodium carboxymethylcellulose as the coating substance and the upper layer of butylacetate-formic acid-water (7:2.5:2.5) as the mobile phase. Apply separately to the plate 10~20 μl of the test solution and 10μl of the reference solution. After developing and removal of the plate, dry it in air, and examine under ultra-violet light (365 nm). The fluorescent spot in the chromatogram obtained with the test solution corresponds in position and colour to the fluorescent spot obtained with the reference solution.

4. Assay

Chlorogenic acid Carry out the method for high performance liquid chromatography (Pharmacopoeia of the People's Republic of China, 2005*ed*).

Chromatographic system and system suitability Use octadecylsilane bonded silica gel as the stationary phase and a mixture of acetonitrile-0.4% phosphoric acid solution (13:87) as the mobile phase. The detection wavelength is 327 nm and the number of theoretical plates of the column is not less than 1000, calculated with reference to the peak of chlorogenic acid.

Reference Preparation Weigh accurately a quantity of chlorogenic acid CRS in an amber coloured volumetric flask, add 50% methanol to produce a solution of 40 μg per ml (Stored at the temperature below 10℃).

Test Preparation Weigh accurately 0.5 g of the powder (through No. 4 sieve) in a conical flask with stopper, add 50 ml of diluted methanol, accurately measured, weigh again and restore the original weight with 50% methanol to the initial weight and mix well. Filter, measure accurately 5 ml of the successive filtrate in a 25 ml amber coloured volumetric flask, add 50% methanol to volume and mix well.

Procedure Inject 5~10 μl of each of the two solutions, accurately measured, into the column. Calculate the content of $C_{16}H_{18}O_9$.

It contains not less than 1.5% of chlorogenic acid ($C_{16}H_{18}O_9$).

Luteolin-7-O-glucoside Carry out the method for high performance liquid chromatography (Pharmacopoeia of the People's Republic of China, 2005*ed*).

Chromatographic system and system suitability Use octadecylsilane bonded silica gel as the stationary phase, acetonitrile as the mobile phase A, 0.5% glacial acetic acid solution as the mobile phase B, elute in gradient as the following:

Time (min)	Mobile phase A (per cent V/V)	Mobile phase B (per cent V/V)
0～30	10→30	90→70

As detector a spectrophotometer set at 350 nm. The number of theoretical plates of the column is not less than 2000, calculated with reference to the peak of luteolin－7－O－glucoside.

Reference Preparation Dissolve a quantity of luteolin－7－O－glucoside CRS, accurately weighed, in 70% ethanol to produce a solution of 40 μg per ml.

Test Preparation Weigh accurately 3 g of the fine powder (through No. 4 sieve) in a conical flask with stopper, add 50 ml of 70% ethanol, accurately measured, weigh and ultrasonic treatment (power, 250 W; frequency, 35 kHz) for 1 hour; cool, weigh again and restore the original weight with 70% ethanol to the initial weight and mix well. Filter and use the successive filtrate as the test solution.

Procedure Inject accurately 10 μl of each of the two solutions into the column and calculate the content.

It contains not less than 0.10 per cent of luteolin－7－O－glucoside ($C_{21}H_{20}O_{11}$), calculated with reference to the dried drug.

Laboratory Assignments

1. Draw the characteristic draft of the powder of Flos Lonecerae Japonicae, and signify glandular hairs, nonglandular hairs and pollens.

2. Look up the documents combine with the results of experiment to draft the stipulation of the quality standard of Flos Lonecerae Japonicae.

Questions

The flower buds of many plants belonging to the same class can be used as Flos Lonicerae. Chinese Pharmacopia (2005 edition) also collects other plants in Caprifoliaceae, including *Lonicera hypoglauca* Miq., *L. confuse* DC. or *L. macranthoides* Hand. -Mazz.. Point out the distinguished characters in the description and microscopic identification between Flos Lonicerae and Flos Lonecerae Japonicae.

实验二十七　菊科生药——红花的鉴定

【实验目的】

1. 掌握红花性状、显微的主要鉴别特征。
2. 掌握红花的化学成分及理化鉴别方法。

【实验材料】

红花 *Carthamus tinctorius* L. 的生药标本；红花药材和粉末。

【实验方法】

1. 性状鉴别

本品为不带子房的管状花，长 1～2 cm。表面黄红色或红色。花冠筒细长，先端 5 裂，裂片狭线形；雄蕊 5 枚，花药聚合成筒状，黄白色；柱头长圆柱形，露出于花药筒外，顶端微分叉。质轻，柔软。气微香，味微苦。

2. 显微鉴别

粉末橙黄色。花冠、花丝、柱头碎片多见，有长管道状分泌细胞，常位于导管旁，直径约至 66 μm，含黄棕色至红棕色分泌物。花粉粒类圆形、椭圆形或橄榄形，直径约至 80 μm,具 3 个萌发孔，外壁有齿状突起。草酸钙方晶存在于薄壁细胞中，直径 2～6 μm。花冠裂片顶端表皮细胞外壁突起呈短绒毛状。柱头及花柱上部细胞分化成圆锥形单细胞毛，先端尖或稍钝。

3. 理化鉴别

（1）取本品 1 g，加稀乙醇 10 ml，振摇浸渍 1 小时，倾取上清液，于浸出液中悬挂一滤纸条，5 分钟后把滤纸条放入水中，片刻取出，滤纸条上部显淡黄色，下部显淡红色。

（2）薄层层析　取红花 0.5 g，加 80% 丙酮溶液 3 ml，密塞，振摇 15 分钟，吸取上清液，作供试品溶液。另取红花对照药材 0.5 g，同法制成对照药材溶液。吸取上述两种溶液点于同一以羧甲基纤维素钠为黏合剂的硅胶 H 薄层板上，以醋酸乙酯－甲酸－水－甲醇（7:2:3:0.4）展开 10 cm，取出，晾干，供试品与对照品显相同的色斑。其中 1 个红色斑点为红花红色素。

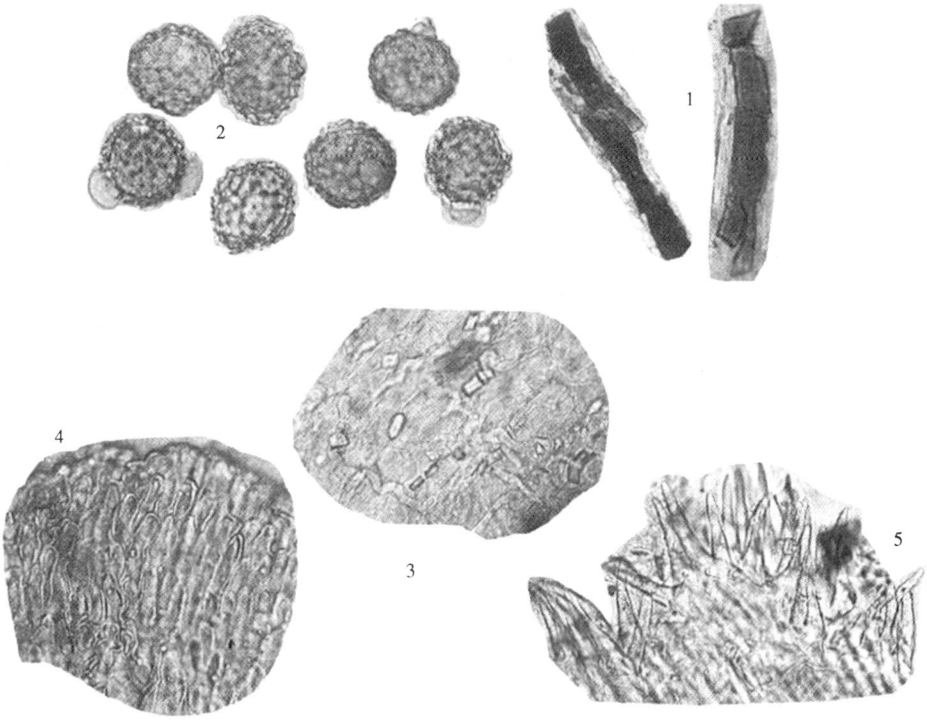

图 27－1　红花粉末

1. 分泌细胞　2. 花粉粒　3. 草酸钙方晶　4. 花冠碎片　5. 柱头碎片

【实验作业】

1. 绘红花花粉粒、柱头上的单细胞非腺毛、含色素管状分泌细胞图。
2. 记述红花理化鉴别的步骤与结果。

【思考题】

1. 花类生药的性状鉴别和显微鉴别的要点有哪些?
2. 采收红花应选择什么样的天气的什么时候? 为什么?

27 Identification of Flos Carthami (Compositae)

Objectives

1. Master the description and microscopic identification of Flos Carthami.

2. Master the chemical constituents and physico-chemical identification on Flos Carthami.

Experiment Material

Crude drug specimens of Flos Carthami; crude drug and powder of Flos Carthami.

Experiment Methods

1. Description

The drug consisting of tubular flowers without ovaries, 1～2 cm long. Externally yellowish-red or red. Corolla tubes slender, 5-lobe at the apex, the lobes narrowly belt-shaped. Staments 5, anthers aggregated to tube, yellowish-white. Stigma long cylindrical, slightly 2-cleft. Texture pliable. Odour, slightly aromatic; taste, slightly bitter.

2. Microscopic identification

Powder orange-yellow. The fragments of corolla, filament and stigma frequently visible. Long tubular secretory cells present generally accompanied by vessels up to 66 μm in diameter, containing yellowish-brown to reddish-brown secretion. Pollen grains subround, elliptical or olivary, up to 80 μm in diameter, with 3 germinal pores, exine dentate-spinose. Prisms of calcium oxalate occurring in parenchymatous cells, 2～6 μm in diameter. Outer walls of terminal epidermal cells of corolla lobes projecting to be tomentellate. Upper epidermal cells of stigma and style differentiated into conical unicellular hairs, acuminate or slightly obtuse at the apex.

3. Physico-chemical identification

(1) Macerate 1 g with 10 ml of dilute ethanol, shake constantly for 1 hour. Decant the supernatant liquid into a beaker, hang a stripe of filter paper in it for 5 minutes, dip the filter paper into water, and immediately take off. The upper part of filter paper shows a pale yellow colour and the lower part stripe shows a pale red colour.

(2) Macerate 0.5 g of the powder with 5 ml of 80% acetone, shake constantly for 15 minutes and allow to stand, the supernatant liquid is used as the test solution. Prepare a solution of Flos Carthami reference drug in the same manner as the reference drug

solution. Carry out the method for thin layer chromatography, using silica gel H containing 0.5% of sodium carboxymethyl cellulose as the coating substance and ethyl acetate-formic acid-water-methanol (7:2:3:0.4) as the mobile phase. Apply separately to the plate 5 μl each of the solutions. After developing and removal of the plate, dry it in air. The spots in the chromatogram obtained with the test solution correspond in position and colour to the spots obtained with the reference drug solution.

Laboratory Assignments

1. Draw the draft of powdered Flos Carthami, including pollens, unicellular non-glandular hairs on the stigma, tubular secretory cells with pigments.

2. Record the procedure and result of physico-chemical identification about Flos Carthami.

Questions

1. What are the main points of description and microscopic identification of flower?

2. Point out the time of weather fitting to gather Flos Carthami, and why?

实验二十八　百部科生药——百部的鉴定

【实验目的】

1. 掌握百部性状、显微的主要鉴别特征。
2. 掌握百部的化学成分及理化鉴别方法。

【实验材料】

直立百部 *Stemona sessilifolia*（Miq.）Miq.、蔓生百部 *S. japonica*（Bl.）Miq. 或对叶百部 *S. tuberosa* Lour. 的生药标本；三种百部的组织切片和百部药材粉末。

【实验方法】

1. 性状鉴别

（1）直立百部　块根纺锤形，上端较细长，有的下端作长尾状，皱缩弯曲，长 4～17 cm，直径 0.5～1 cm。表面黄白色或土黄色，有不规则深纵沟，间或有横皱纹。质脆，受潮后软韧，断面平坦，角质样，淡黄棕色或黄白色，皮部宽广，中柱扁缩。气微，味甘、苦。

（2）蔓生百部　根两端狭细，长 3～10 cm，直径约 1 cm。表面淡灰白色，多不规则皱褶，有的可见横皱纹。

（3）对叶百部　纺锤形或长条形，长 8～24 cm，直径 0.8～2 cm。表面淡黄棕色或灰棕色，具浅纵皱纹或不规则纵槽。质坚实，断面黄白色或暗棕色，中柱较大，髓部类白色。

2. 显微鉴别

（1）直立百部根横切面：根被为 3～4 列细胞，壁木栓化及木化，具致密的细条纹。皮层较宽。中柱韧皮部束与木质部束各 19～27 个，间隔排列，韧皮部束内侧有少数非木化纤维；木质部束导管 2～5 个，并有木纤维及管胞，导管类多角形，径向直径约至 48 μm，偶有导管深入至髓部。髓部散有少数细小纤维。

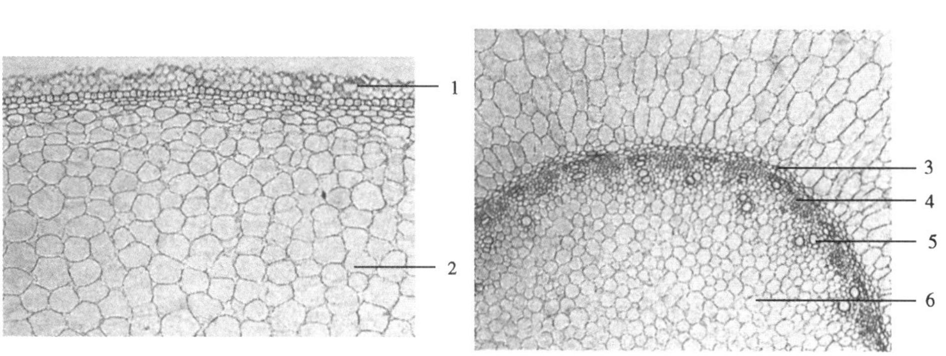

图 28－1　直立百部（根）横切面

1. 根被　2. 皮层　3. 内皮层　4. 韧皮部　5. 木质部　6. 髓

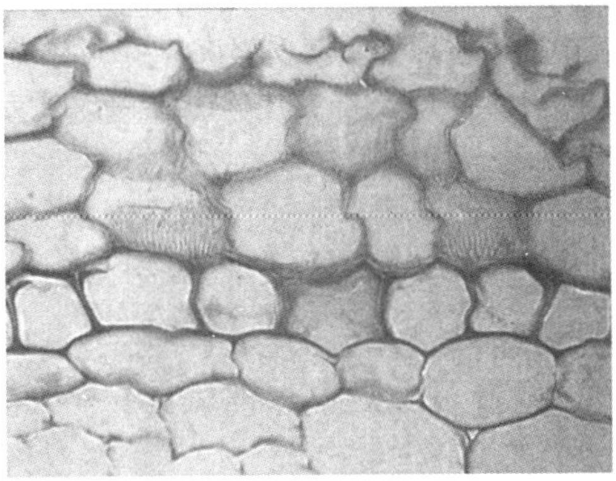

图 28－2　根被

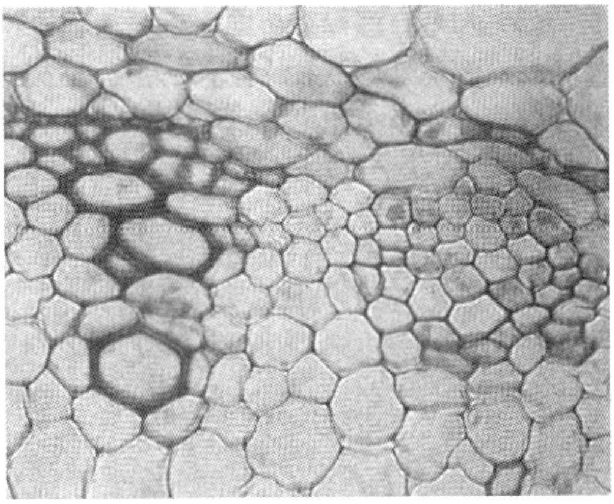

图 28－3　韧皮部束和木质部束

(2) 蔓生百部根横切面：根被为 3～6 列细胞。韧皮部纤维木化。导管径向直径约至 184 μm，通常深入至髓部，与外侧导管束作 2～3 轮排列。

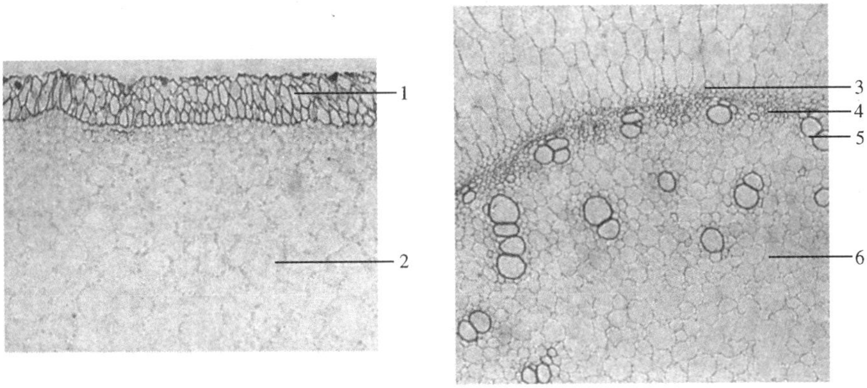

图 28－4　蔓生百部（根）横切面

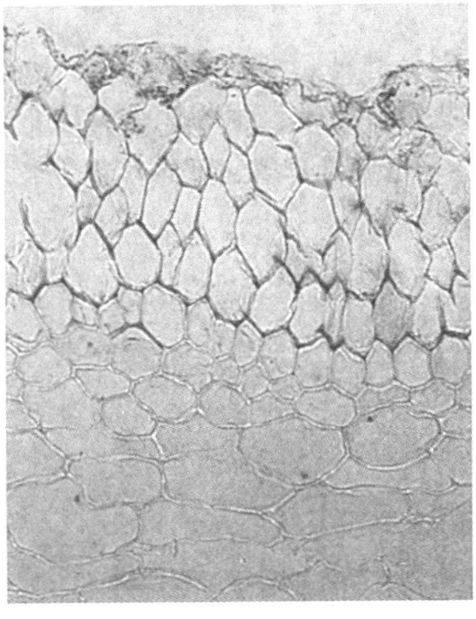

图 28－5　根被

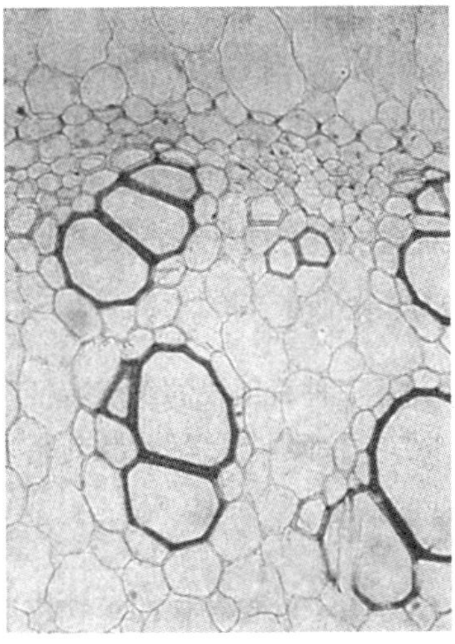

图 28－6　韧皮部束和木质部束

（3）对叶百部根横切面：根被细胞为3列细胞，细胞壁无细条纹，其最内层细胞的内壁特厚。皮层外侧散有纤维，类方形，壁微木化。中柱木质部束和韧皮部束各32～40个。木质部束导管圆多角形，直径至107 μm，其内侧与木纤维及微木化的薄壁细胞连接成环层。

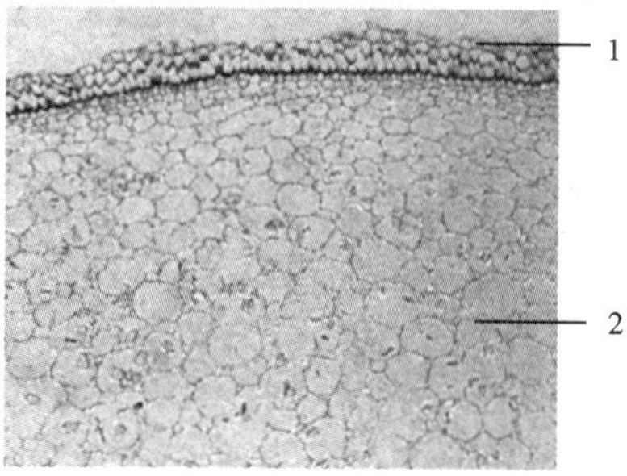

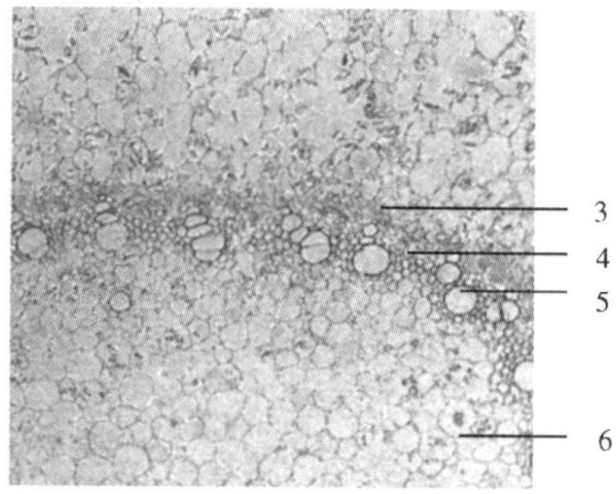

图28－7　对叶百部（根）横切面

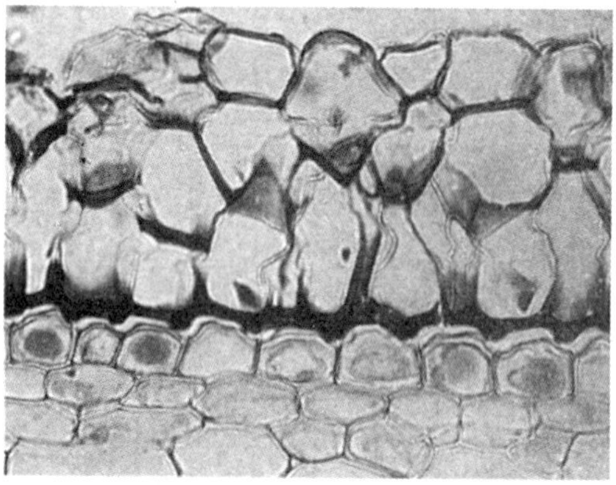

图28－8　根被

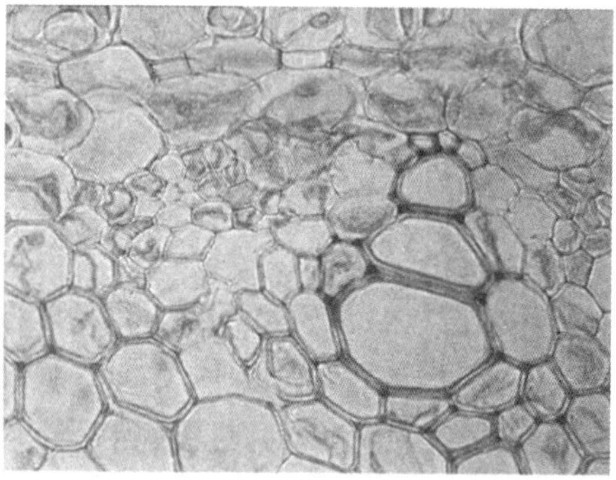

图28－9　韧皮部束和木质部束

3. 理化鉴别

取粉末5 g，加70%乙醇50 ml，加热回流1小时，过滤，滤液蒸去乙醇，残渣加浓氨试液调节pH至10～11，再加三氯甲烷5 ml振摇提取，分取三氯甲烷层，蒸干，残渣加1%盐酸溶液5 ml使溶解，滤过。滤液分为两份：一份中滴加碘化铋钾试液，生成橙红色沉淀；另一份中滴加硅钨酸试液，生成乳白色沉淀。

【实验作业】

1. 记述三种百部根的组织特征与区别点，并绘直立百部根的组织简图。
2. 记录百部理化鉴别步骤与结果。

【思考题】

1. 试述单子叶植物根的组织构造。
2. 百部主含何种化学成分、如何鉴别?

28 Identification of Radix Stemonae (Stemonaceae)

Objectives

1. Master the description and microscopic identification of Radix Stemonae.

2. Master the chemical constituents and physico-chemical identification of Radix Stemonae.

Experiment Material

Crude drug specimens from *Stemona seessilifolia* (Miq.) Miq., *S. japonica* (Bl.) Miq. or *S. tuberosa* Lour. Permanent mounts of 3 species from Genus *Stemon*a, powdered Radix Stemonae.

Experiment Methods

1. Description

Root of *Stemona sessilitfolia* Fusiform. The upper end relatively slender, shrunken and curved, 4 ~ 17 cm long, 0.5 ~ 1 cm in diameter. Externally yellowish-white or pale brownish-yellow, with irregular longitudinal deep furrows, and occasionally transverse wrinkles. Texture fragile, easily broken, fracture even, horny, pale yellowish-brown or yellowish-white, bark broad, stele compressed. Odour, slight; taste, sweet and bitter.

Root of *Stemona japonica* Two ends slightly thinned, 3 ~ 10 cm long. Externally mostly with irregular longitudinal folds and transverse wrinkle.

Root of *Stemona tuberosa* Long fusiform or long slatshaped, 8 ~ 24 cm long, 0.8 ~ 2 cm in diameter. Externally yellowish-brown to greyish-brown, with shallow longitudinal wrinkles or irregular longitudinal furrows. Texture compact, fracture yellowish-white or dark brown, stele large, pith whitish.

2. Microscopic identification

Transverse section:

Root of *Stemona sessilitfolia* Velamen of 3 ~ 4 layers of cells, walls suberized and lignified with dense and fine striations. Cortex relatively broad. In stele phloem bundles and xylem bundles 19 ~ 27, respectively, arranged alternatively, with a few non-lignified fibres in the inner side of phloem bundles; xylem bundles with 2 ~ 5 vessels, xylem fibres and tracheids, vessels subpolygonal, 48 μm in diameter, radially, occasionally penetrating into the pith. A few small fibres scattered in pith.

Root of *Stemona japonica* Velamen of 3 ~ 6 layers of cells. Phloem fibres lignified. Vessels up to 184 μm in diameter, radially, usually penetrating into pith, arranged in 2~3 whorls.

Root of *Stemona tuberose* Velamen of 3 layers of cells, walls without fine striations, the inner walls of the inner layers heavily thickened. Fibres scattered in the outer part of cortex, subsquare, with slightly lignified walls. In stele xylem bundles and phloem bundles 32~40 respectively. Vessels in xylem bundles rounded polygonal, up to 107 μm in diameter. The inner sides of xylem bundles linked up with xylem fibres and slightly lignified parenchymatous cells into a ring.

3. Physico-chemical identification

Heat under reflux 5 g of the powder with 50 ml of 70% ethanol for 1 hour, filter, and evaporate the filtrate for removing ethanol. To the residue add strong ammonia TS, adjust to pH 10 ~ 11, extract by shaking with 5 ml of chloroform. Evaporate the chloroform solution to dryness, dissolve the residue in 5 ml of 1% hydrochloric acid solution and filter. Divide the filtrate into two portions. To one portion add 1 drop of bismuth potassium iodide TS, an orange-red precipitate is produced; to another portion add 1 drop of silicotungstic acid TS, a miky-white precipitate is produced.

Laboratory Assignments

1. State the tissue characters of 3 species from Genus *Stemona*, point out the distinguishing characters of them and make a diagram of the transverse section from *Stemona seessilifolia*.

2. Record the procedure and result of physico-chemical identification on Radix Stemonae.

Questions

1. Try to state the tissue structure of root from monocotyledon.

2. What kind of chemical constituents are contained in Radix Stemonae and how to identify them?

实验二十九　百合科生药——川贝母、浙贝母的鉴定

【实验目的】

1. 掌握川贝母与浙贝母的性状、显微的主要鉴别特征。
2. 掌握川贝母与浙贝母的化学成分及理化鉴别方法。
3. 了解同属植物贝母类生药的鉴别特征。

【实验材料】

川贝母 *Fritillaria cirrhosa* D.Don、暗紫贝母 *F.unibracteata* Hsiao et K.C.Hsia、甘肃贝母 *F.przewalskii* Maxim. 或梭砂贝母 *F.delavayi* Franch. 的生药标本（其按性状不同习称："松贝"、"青贝"），川贝母粉末；浙贝母 *F.thunbergii* Miq. 的生药标本（其按大小习称："大贝"、"珠贝"），浙钡母粉末。

【实验方法】

1. 性状鉴别

（1）松贝：呈类圆锥形或近球形，高 0.3～0.8 cm，直径 0.3～0.9 cm。表面类白色；外层两枚鳞叶大小悬殊，大鳞叶紧裹小鳞叶，未抱部分呈新月形，习称"怀中抱月"，顶端闭合，内有类圆柱形、顶端稍尖的心芽和小鳞叶 1～2 枚；先端钝圆或稍尖，底部平，微凹入，中心有 1 灰褐色的鳞茎盘，偶有残存须根。质硬而脆，断面白色，富粉性。气微。味微苦。

（2）青贝：呈类扁球形，高 0.4～1.4 cm，直径 0.4～1.6 cm。外层两枚鳞叶大小相近，相对抱合，顶端开裂，内有心芽和小鳞叶 2～3 枚及细圆柱形的残茎。

（3）大贝：为鳞茎外层的单瓣鳞叶，略呈新月形，高 1～2 cm，直径 2～3.5 cm。外表面灰白色至淡黄色，内表面白色或淡棕色，被白色粉末。质硬脆，易折断，断面白色或黄白色，富粉性。气微，味微苦。

（4）珠贝：为完整的鳞茎，扁圆形，高 1～1.5 cm，直径 1～2.5 cm。表面类白色，外层 2 枚鳞叶，肥厚，略呈肾形，相对抱合，中央有 2～3 枚小鳞叶及干缩的残茎。

2. 显微鉴别

（1）川贝母：淀粉粒单粒大多呈广卵形、长圆形或不规则形，有的边缘不平整或略作分枝状，直径 5～64 μm；脐点大多不明显，细点状或短缝状；层纹隐约可见。表皮细胞类长方形，垂周壁波状弯曲，偶见不定式气孔，圆形或扁圆形。

（2）浙贝母：淀粉粒众多，单粒长卵形、广卵形或椭圆形，直径 5～56 μm；脐点点状、裂缝状、人字状，位于较小端，层纹大多明显；复粒与半复粒稀少，复粒由 2～3 分粒组成。表皮细胞表面观类多角形或长方形，垂周壁连珠状增厚；有的可见气孔。

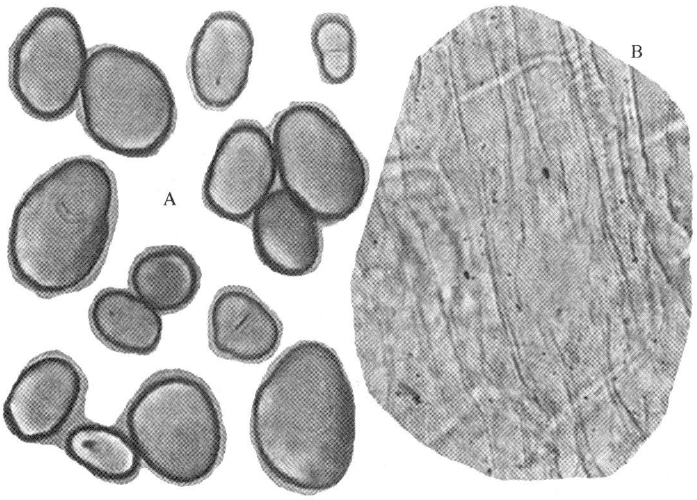

图 29－1　川贝母粉末

A. 淀粉粒　　B. 表皮细胞

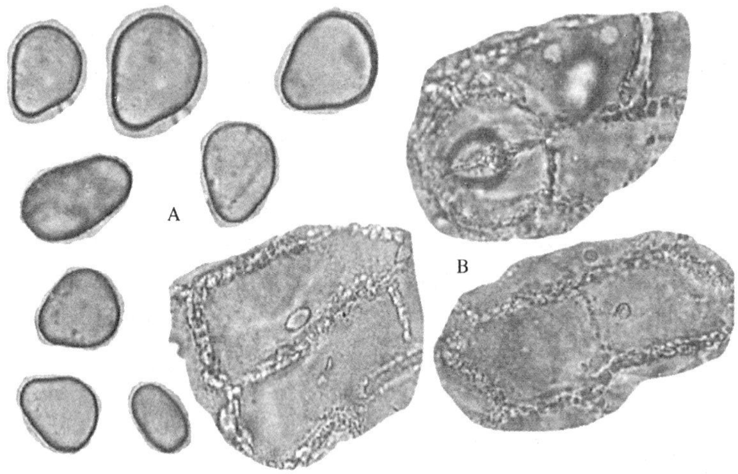

图 29－2　浙贝母粉末

A. 淀粉粒　　B. 表皮细胞

3. 理化鉴别

（1）取样品粉末 1 g，加 70％的乙醇 20 ml，加热回流 30 分钟，过滤，滤液蒸干，残渣加三氯甲烷 1 ml 使溶解，滤过，取滤液分置两支试管中，一支加 3 滴碘化铋钾试液，生成橘红色沉淀；另一支加 1～3 滴硅钨酸试液，产生白色絮状沉淀。

（2）薄层层析：取样品粉末 10 g，加浓氨溶液 2.0 ml 与三氯甲烷 20 ml，涡旋，过夜，滤过。滤液蒸干，残渣加三氯甲烷 0.5 ml 溶解，作供试品溶液。另取贝母碱、异贝母碱、去氢贝母碱、西贝素、川贝酮、平贝碱甲加三氯甲烷溶解制成约每毫升含 0.5 mg 的溶液，作对照品溶液。以上溶液分别点样于硅胶 GF_{254} 薄层板，以醋酸乙酯－甲醇－浓氨溶液(85∶10∶5)展开。取出，晾干，用改良碘化铋钾试液显色，供试品色谱在与对照品色谱的相应位置上显相同棕黄色斑点。

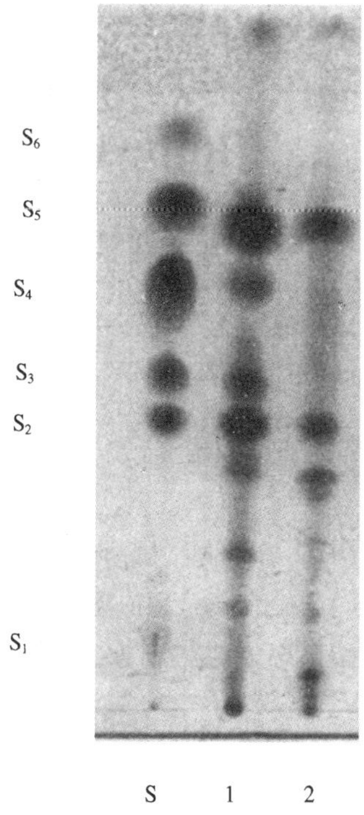

图 29－3　贝母薄层层析图谱

1. 浙贝母（*Fritillaria thunbergii* Miq.）2. 川贝母（*Fritillaria cirrhosa* D.Don）

S_1. 平贝碱甲　S_2. 贝母碱　S_3. 异贝母碱　S_4. 西贝素　S_5. 去氢贝母碱　S_6. 川贝酮

(3) DNA 分子遗传标记鉴定：贝母鳞茎（或叶）适量，按 DNA 提取方法提取模板 DNA，以 5SrRNA 为引物进行 PCR 扩增。PCR 产物分别进行克隆、测序或酶解，结果表明：川贝母和浙贝母的 5SrRNA 空间区的 DNA 序列区别明显，与其他贝母比较，川贝母在 22～35 和230～240 的序列是特有的，而在 130～135 的序列与浙贝母等其他贝母不同。二者的 *EcoR* Ⅰ 酶切位点也区别明显。

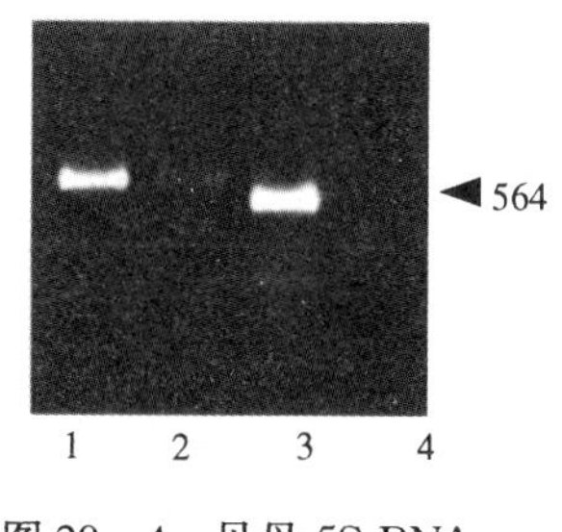

图 29－4　贝母 5SrRNA 空间区基因酶解产物电泳图谱

1. *Fritillaria puqiensis*
2. *F. anhuiensis*
3. *F. thunbergii*
4. *F. cirrhosa*

【实验作业】

1. 分别绘川贝母、浙贝母粉末显微特征图，并简述两者的鉴别点。

2. 记述理化鉴别步骤与结果。

【思考题】

如何从性状特征上区别川贝母与浙贝母？

29 Identification of Bulbus Fritillariae Cirrhosae and Bulbus Fritillariae Thunbergii (Liliaceae)

Objectives

1. Master the description and identification of Bulbus Fritillariae Cirrhosae and Bulbus Fritilllariae Thunbergii.

2. Master the chemical constituents and physico-chemical identification on Bulbus Fritillariae Cirrhosae and Bulbus Fritilllariae Thunbergii.

3. Study the characters of different species from Genus *Fritillaria*.

Experiment Material

Crude drug specimens of *Fritillaria cirrhosa* D.Don, *F. unibracteata* Hsiao et K.C.Hsia, *F. przewalskii* Maxim., *F. delavayi* Franch., *Fritilllaria thunbergii* Miq., and their powder.

Experiment Methods

1. Description

Songbei: Subconical or subspherical, 0.3 ~ 0.8 cm high, 0.3 ~ 0.9 cm in diameter. Externally whitish. The outer scale leaves 2, varying considerably in size, with the large scale closely embracing the small one, the uncovered part appearing crescent, commonly known as "Huaizhong Baoyue" (holding the moon in the arms). Apex closed, with subcylinerical and slightly acute, base even and slightly concave, with a greyish-brown disk at central part, remains of fibrous roots occasionally found. Texture hard and fragile, fracture white, starchy, Odour, slight; taste, slightly bitter.

Qingbei: Nearly oblate, 0.4 ~ 1.4 cm high, 0.4 ~ 1.6 cm in diameter. Outer scale leaves 2, almost uniform in size, embraced. Apex open, with buds and 2 ~ 3 small scales inside and slender cylindrical remains of a stem.

Dabei: The outer single scale leaf of bulb, almost in crescent shape, 1 ~ 2 cm high, 2 ~ 3.5 cm in diameter. The outer surface whitish to pale yellow, the inner surface white or pale brown, covered with white powder. Texture hard and fragile, easily broken, fracture white to yellowish-white, highly starchy. Odour, slight; taste, slightly bitter.

Zhubei: Whole bulb, oblate, 1～1.5 cm high, 1～2.5 cm in diameter. Externally whitish, the outer scale leaves 2, plump and fleshy, slightly in reniform, holding to each other, containing 2～3 small scale leaves and dried shrunken stem remains.

2. Microscopic identification

Chuanbeimu: Starch granules fairly abundant, broadly ovoid, long spheroidal or irregularly spheroidal, some with uneven or slightly branch-like edges, 5～64 μm in diameter, hilum short slit-shaped or pointed and faint striations visible. Epidermal cells subrectangular, anticlinal walls sinuous, rounded or oblate anomocytic stomata occasionally found.

Zhebeimu: Starch granules numerous, simple granules ovoid, broad-ovoid or elliptical, 5～56 μm in diameter, hilum pointed, cleft-like or V-shaped in the smaller end, striations mostly distinct; semi-compound and compound granules rare, compound-granules composed of 2～3 components visible occasionally. Epidermal cells subpolygonal or rectangular, anticlinal walls beaded-thickened; Stomata sometimes visible.

3. Physico-chemical identification

(1) Heat under reflux 1 g of the coarse powder with 20 ml of 70% ethanol for about 30 minutes, filter and evaporate to dryness. Dissolve the residue in 1 ml of chloroform, filter and transfer the filtrate to two test tubes respectively. To one tube add 3 drops of potassium iodobismuthate TS, an orange precipitate is produced; to another tube add 1～3 drops of silicotungstic acid TS; a white flocculent precipitate is produced.

(2) TLC: To 10 g of the powder add 2.0 ml of ammonia solution and 20 ml of chloroform, mix well, allow to stand overnight, filter and evaporate to dryness. Dissolve the residue in 0.5 ml of chloroform, as the test solutions. To verticine, isoverticine, verticinone, sipeimine, chuanbeinone and pinpeimine, dissolve with an appropriate quantity of chloroform (0.5 mg/ml), as the reference solutions. Pipette them respectively, spot on the same TLC plate (silica gel GF_{254}), mobile phase: ethyl acetate-methanol-strong ammonia solution (85∶10∶5), after developing and removal of the plate, dry it in air, spray with dilute potassium iodobismuthate TS, the principal spot in the chromatogram obtained with the test solution correspond to the color and position with the principal spot obtained with the reference solution.

(3) DNA molecule genetic marker: some bulbs or leaves from Genus *Fritillaria*, extract template DNA as usual, PCR amplification from 5SrRNA. Clone, sequencing and enzymolysis PCR product, the results indicate: DNA zone of 5SrRNA of Bulbus Fritillariae Cirrhosae and Bulbus Fritillariae Thunbergii are different evidently, compare to other Fritillariae, 22～35 sequence and 230～240 sequence of Bulbus Fritillariae Cirrhosae is characteristic, and its 130～135 sequence is different from other

Fritillaria. Their *EcoR* Ⅰ enzyme sites also are different obviously.

Laboratory Assignments

1. Make drawings of power of Bulbus Fritillariae Cirrhosae and Bulbus Fritillariae Thunbergii respectively, and record the distinguishing characters of them.

2. Record the procedure and result of physico-chemical identification.

Questions

How to differ Bulbus Fritillariae Cirrhosae from Bulbus Fritillariae Thunbergii in their description?

实验三十　百合科生药——麦冬的鉴定

【实验目的】

1. 掌握麦冬性状、显微的主要鉴别特征。
2. 掌握麦冬的化学成分及理化鉴别方法。

【实验材料】

麦冬 *Ophiopogon japonicus*（Thunb.）Ker-Gawl. 的药材，湖北麦冬 *Liriope spicata*（Thunb.）Lour. var. *prolifera* Y.T. Ma 的药材。

【实验方法】

1. 性状鉴别

（1）麦冬：块根呈纺锤形，两端略尖，长 1.5～3.5 cm，直径 3～7 mm。表面黄白色或淡黄色，有细纵纹。质硬韧，断面类白色，半透明，中柱细小。气微香，味甘、微苦。

（2）湖北麦冬：块根呈纺锤形，长 1.2～4 cm，直径 4～9 mm；表面类黄色，半透明。质硬脆，断面类黄色，角质样。微香，味甘。

2. 显微鉴别

分别取上述两种药材，作徒手切片，并进行如下观察。

（1）麦冬块根横切面：表皮细胞 1 列，根被为 2～5 列木化细胞。皮层宽广，散有含草酸钙针晶束的黏液细胞；内皮层细胞壁均匀增厚，木化，有通道细胞，外侧为 1 列石细胞，其内壁及侧壁增厚，纹孔细密。中柱较小，韧皮部束 15～24 个，各位于木质部束的星角间。髓小，薄壁细胞类圆形。

（2）湖北麦冬块根横切面：表皮细胞 1 列。皮层宽广；外皮层细胞 1 列，间有分泌细胞；靠接内皮层的 1 列细胞，内壁及侧壁增厚；内皮层细胞侧壁增厚或侧壁及内壁增厚，木化。中柱木质部束及韧皮部束各 8～14 个。髓细胞非木化。

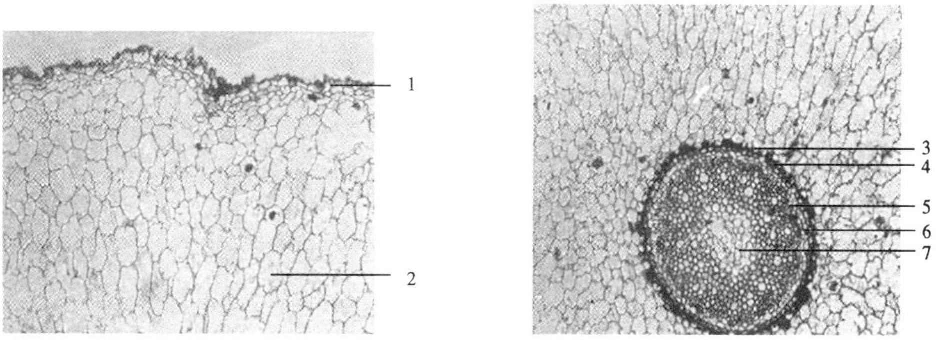

图 30－1　麦冬（块根）横切面

1. 根被　2. 皮层　3. 石细胞　4. 内皮层　5. 韧皮部　6. 木质部　7. 髓

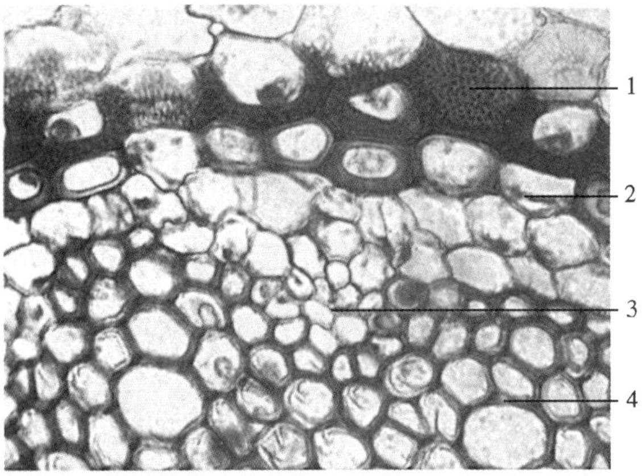

图 30－2　中柱

1. 石细胞　2. 内皮层　3. 韧皮部　4. 木质部

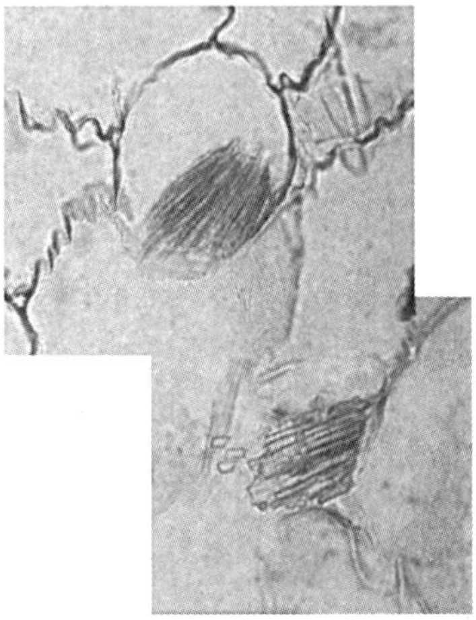

图 30－3　草酸钙针晶

3. 理化鉴别

取麦冬薄片，置紫外灯（365 nm）下观察，显浅蓝色荧光。

【实验作业】

1. 记述麦冬与湖北麦冬的异同点。
2. 绘麦冬根的组织简图。

【思考题】

1. 什么叫通道细胞？
2. 商品麦冬的原植物来源，除了麦冬、湖北麦冬外，还有哪些，如何鉴别？

30 Identification of Radix Ophiopogonis (Liliaceae)

Objectives

1. Master the description and microscopoic identification of Radix Ophiopogonis.

2. Master the chemical constituents and physico-chemical identification on Radix Ophiopogonis.

Experiment Material

Crude drug specimens of *Ophiopogon japonicus* (Thunb.) Ker-Gawl and *Liriope spicata* (Thunb.) Lour. var. *prolifera* Y. T. Ma.

Experiment Methods

1. Description

(1) *Ophiopogon japonicus*: Fusiform with two ends slightly tapering, 1.5~3.5 cm long, 3~7 mm in diameter; externally yellowish-white. Finely wrinkled longitudinally. Texture tough. Fracture yellowish-white, translucent, stele small. Odour slightly aromatic, taste, sweetish and bitterish.

(2) *Liriope spicata* var. *prolifera*: Root tuber is fusiform, 1.2~4 cm long, 4~9 mm in diameter; externally yellowish, translucent. Texture hard and fragile after drying, fracture pale-yellow, horny. Odour, slight; taste, sweet.

2. Microscopic identification

Take these two drugs, cut into slices by hands, and observe the characters.

(1) Transverse section of the root from *O. japonicus*: Epidermis consisting of 1 layer of cells. Velamen of 2~5 layers of lignified cells. Cortex broad, scattered with mucilage cells containing raphides of calcium oxalate. Endodermal cells with evently thickened and lignified walls, and endodermis with passage cells, the outside of endodermis lying a layer of stone cells, the inner and lateral walls thickened. Finely and close pitted. Stele relatively small. Phloem bundles 15~24, located between the xylem arms. Pith small, parenchymatous cells subround.

(2) Transverse section of the root from *Liriope spicata* var. *prolifera*: Epidermis consisting of 1 layer of cells. Cortex broad, exodermis consisting of 1 layer cells, with secretory cells, endodermal cells with thickened and lignified walls, stele phloem bundles

and xylem bundles 8～14 respectively. The cells of pith is unlignified.

3. Physico-chemical identification

Examine a thin slice of the drug under ultra-violet light (365 nm) a pale blue fluorescence is produced.

Laboratory Assignments

1. Point out the distinguishing characters of *O. japonicus* and *L. spicata* var. *prolifera*.
2. Make a diagram of the transverse section of *O. japonicus*.

Questions

1. What is passage cell?
2. Write out the sources about original plant of commodity Maidong except *O. japonicus* and *L. spicata* var. *prolifera*. How to identify them?

实验三十一　姜科生药——砂仁的鉴定

【实验目的】

1．掌握砂仁性状、显微的主要鉴别特征。
2．掌握砂仁的化学成分及理化鉴别方法。
3．掌握砂仁的挥发油含量测定方法。

【实验材料】

阳春砂 *Amomum villosum* Lour．的生药标本、种子组织切片及药材粉末。

【实验方法】

1．性状鉴别

阳春砂　呈椭圆形或卵圆形，有不明显的三棱，长 1.5～2.5 cm，直径 1～2 cm。表面棕褐色，密生刺状突起，顶端有花被残基，基部常有果梗。果皮薄而软。种子集结成团，具三钝棱，中有白色隔膜，将种子团分成 3 瓣，每瓣有种子 5～26 粒。种子为不规则多面体，直径 2～3 mm；表面棕红色或暗褐色，有细皱纹，外被淡棕色膜质假种皮；质硬，胚乳灰白色。气芳香而浓烈，味辛凉、微苦。

2．显微鉴别

（1）阳春砂种子横切面：假种皮有时残存；种皮表皮 1 列，径向延长，壁稍厚；下皮细胞 1 列，含棕色或红棕色物；油细胞层为 1 列油细胞，长 76～106 μm，宽 16～25 μm，含黄色油滴；色素层为数列棕色细胞，细胞多角形，排列不规则；内种皮为 1 列栅状厚壁细胞，黄棕色，内壁及侧壁极厚，细胞小，内含硅质块；外胚乳细胞和内胚乳细胞均含淀粉粒。

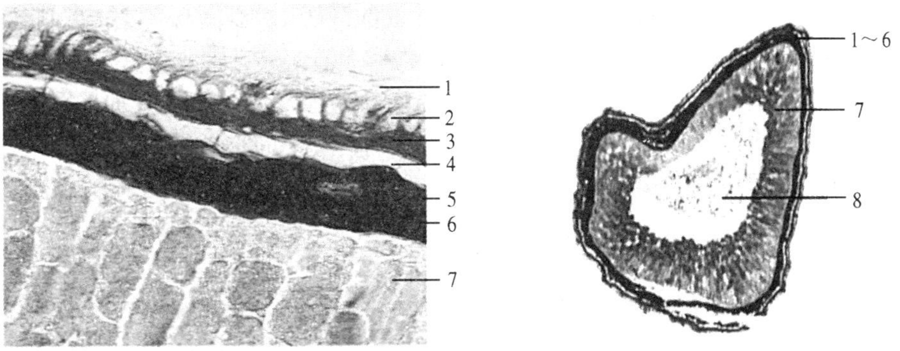

图 31－1　阳春砂种子横切面

1．假种皮　2．种皮表皮　3．下皮　4．油细胞层　5．色素层　6．内种皮　7．胚乳　8．胚

(2) 粉末灰棕色。

①内种皮厚壁细胞红棕色或黄棕色，表面观多角形，壁厚，非木化，胞腔内含硅质块；断面观为1列栅状细胞，内壁及侧壁极厚，胞腔偏外侧，内含硅质块。

②种皮表皮细胞淡黄色，表面观长条形，常与下皮细胞上下层垂直排列。

③下皮细胞含棕色或红棕色物。

此外，尚可见色素层细胞、外胚乳和内胚乳细胞、淀粉粒、油细胞等。

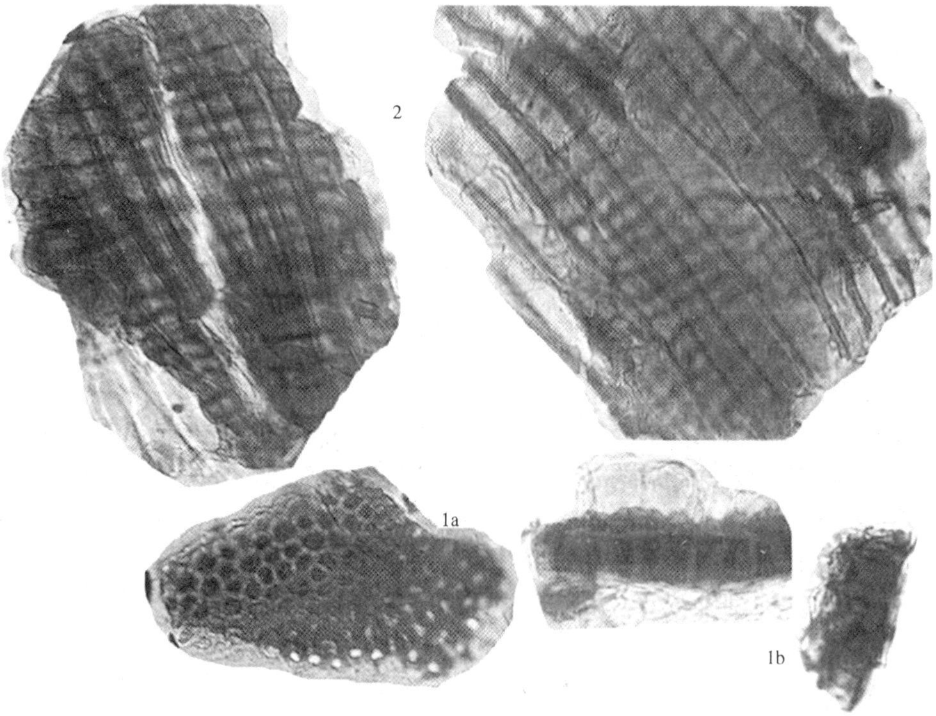

图 31－2　砂仁粉末

1. 内种皮细胞（a. 表面观　b. 侧面观）　2. 种皮表皮与下皮细胞

3. 理化鉴别

提取本品挥发油，加乙醇制成每1 ml含20 μl的溶液，作供试品溶液。另取醋酸龙脑酯对照品，加乙醇制成每1 ml含10 μl的溶液，作对照品溶液。吸取上述两种溶液各1 μl，分别点于同一硅胶G薄层板上，以环己烷－醋酸乙酯（22∶1）为展开剂，展开，取出，晾干，喷5%香草醛硫酸溶液，加热至斑点显色清晰。供试品色谱中，在与对照品色谱相应位置上，显相同的紫红色斑点。

4. 含量测定

照挥发油测定法测定。一般规定阳春砂、绿壳砂种子团含挥发油不得少于3.0%（ml/g）；海南砂种子团含挥发油不得少于1.0%（ml/g）。

【实验作业】

1. 绘阳春砂种子横切面组织简图和粉末显微特征图，示内种皮厚壁细胞、种皮表皮及下皮细胞。

2. 记录理化鉴别步骤，并绘制薄层色谱图。

3. 记录含量测定步骤及结果。

【思考题】

1. 种子类生药的性状鉴别和显微鉴别有哪些要点?

2. 除阳春砂外，《中国药典》还收载了哪些来源的砂仁？还有哪些植物的果实在部分地区作砂仁用?

31 Identification of Fructus Amomi (Zingiberaceae)

Objectives

1. Master the description and microscopic identification of Fructus Amomi.

2. Master the chemical constituents and physico-chemical identification on Fructus Amomi.

3. Master the method for determination of volatile oil on Fructus Amomi.

Experiment Material

Crude drug specimens from *Amomum villosum* Lour.; Permanent mounts of Fructus Amomi; Powdered Fructus Amomi.

Experiment Methods

1. Description

Fruit of *Amomum villosum* ellipsoidal or ovoid, indistinctly 3-ridged, 1.5~2.5 cm long, 1 ~ 2 cm in diameter. Externally brown, densely covered with spiny protrudings, apex with remains of perianth, and base often bearing a fruit stalk. Pericarp thin and soft. Seeds agglutinated into a mass, 3-ridged obtusely, divided into 3 groups by white septa, and each group containing 5~26 seeds. Seeds irregularly polyhedral, 2 ~ 3 mm in diameter; externally brownish-red or dark brown, finely wrinkled, covered with pale brown membranous aril; texture hard, endosperm greyish-white. Odour, strongly aromatic; taste, pungent, cool and slightly bitter.

2. Microscopic identification

(1) Transverse section of seed from *Amomum villosum*: sometimes remains of aril present. Epidermal cells of testa 1 row, radially elongated, slightly thick-walled; hypodermal cells 1 row, containing brown or reddish-brown contents. Oil cells in 1 row 76~ 100 μm long, 16 ~ 25 μm wide, containing yellow oil droplets. Pigment layer consisting of several rows of brown cells, polygonal, and irregularly arranged. Endotesta consisting 1 row of palisade-like thick-walled cell, yellowish-brown, small, with heavily thickened inner and lateral walls, containing a silica body. Cell of perisperm and Cell of endosperm containing starch granules.

(2) Powder: Greyish-brown.

① Thick-walled cells of endotesta reddish-brown or yellowish-brown, polygonal in surface view, with thickened and non-lignified walls, lumen containing a silica body; showing 1 row of palisade cells in section view with heavily thickened inner and lateral walls, lumen inclined to the outer side and containing a silica body.

② Epidermal cells of testa pale yellow, stripe-shaped in surface view, usually vertically arranged with hypodermal cells in an upper and lower layered pattern.

③ Hypodermal cells containing brown or reddish-brown contents.

④ Cells of pigment layer; cells of perisperm, cells of endosperm, starch grains and oil cells can be seen.

3. Physico-chemical identification

Dissolve the volatile oil in ethanol to produce a solution containing 20 μl per ml as the test solution. Dissolve bornyl acetate CRS in ethanol to produce a solution containing 10 μl per ml as the reference solution. Using silica gel G as the coating substance and a mixture of cyclohexane-ethyl acetate (22∶1) as the mobile phase. Apply separately to the plate 1 μl of each of the two solutions. After developing and removal of the plate, dry it in air, spray with a 5% solution of vanillin in sulfuric acid, heat until the color of the spot cleared up. A purplish-red spot in the chromatogram obtained with the test solution corresponds in position and color to the spot in the chromatogram obtained with the reference solution.

4. Assay

Carry out the method for the determination of volatile oil. Masses of seeds of *Amomum villosum* and *A. villosum* var. *xanthioides* contain not less than 3.0% of volatile oil (ml/g); masses of seed of *Amomum longiligulare* contain not less than 1.0% of volatile oil (ml/g) .

Laboratory Assignments

1. Make diagrams of transverse section and powder from Fructus Amomi, and show the thick-walled cells of endotesta, epidermal cells of testa and hypodermal cells.

2. Record the procedure of physico-chemical identification and make a chart of TLC.

3. Note the procedure and result of assay.

Questions

1. What are the key points of description identification and microscopic identification for semen drugs?

2. What are the other Fructus Amomi included in Pharmacopoeia of the People's Republic of China besides *Amomum vilosum* Lour.,? What other fruits of plants are used as Fructus Amomi locally?

实验三十二　兰科生药——天麻的鉴定

【实验目的】

1. 掌握天麻性状、显微的主要鉴别特征。
2. 掌握天麻的化学成分及理化鉴别方法。
3. 了解天麻的常见伪品在性状、显微特征上与天麻的主要区别。

【实验材料】

天麻 *Gastrodia elata* Bl. 的生药标本；天麻块茎组织切片及天麻药材粉末。

【实验方法】

1. 性状鉴别

块茎长椭圆形，稍扁缩弯曲，长 3～15 cm，宽 1.5～6 cm，厚 0.5～2 cm。表面黄白色至黄褐色，多不规则纵皱纹，有由潜伏芽排列成的多轮横环纹，有时可见棕黑色菌丝。顶端有红棕色鹦哥嘴状顶芽（冬麻），或残留有茎基（春麻），末端有圆脐形疤痕。质坚实，断面较平坦，黄白色或淡棕色，角质样。气微，味甘。

2. 显微鉴别

（1）天麻块茎横切面：表皮有时残存；下皮为 2～3 列切向延长的木栓化细胞。皮层为 10 数列多角形细胞，有的含草酸钙针晶束。较老块茎外侧皮层为 2～3 列厚壁细胞，壁木化，有纹孔。中柱大，周韧型维管束散列；薄壁细胞含草酸钙针晶束。

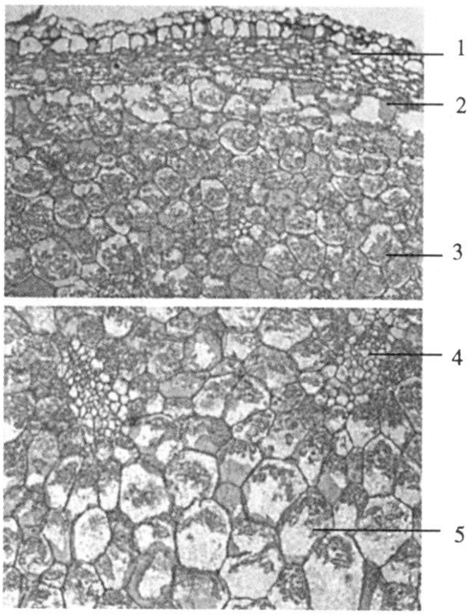

图 32－1　天麻（块茎）横切面

1. 下皮　2. 皮层　3. 中柱　4. 维管束　5. 髓

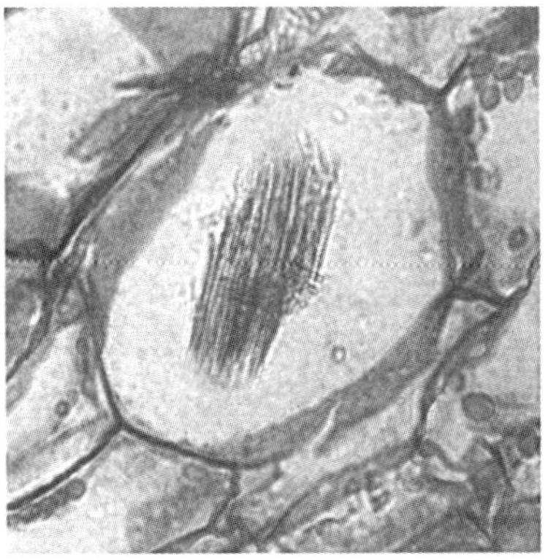

图 32-2　草酸钙针晶

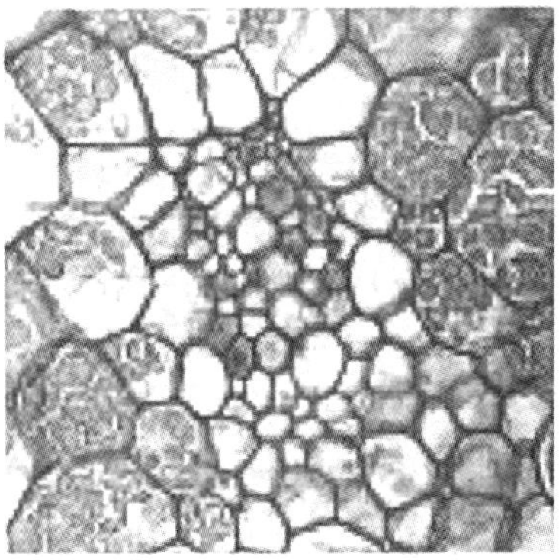

图 32-3　维管束

（2）粉末：黄白色至黄棕色。①用醋酸甘油水装片观察含糊化多糖类物。薄壁细胞无色，有的角质样，有条纹；有的细胞可见长卵形或类圆形颗粒（颗粒清晰与否，与蒸煮加工糊化程度有关），遇碘液显棕色或淡棕紫色。② 草酸钙针晶成束或散在，长 25～75 (93) μm。③厚壁细胞表面观呈多角形或类椭圆形，纹孔明显。④薄壁细胞淡黄棕色，大多皱缩，有的细胞形大，壁稍增厚，非木化，纹孔较大而密。

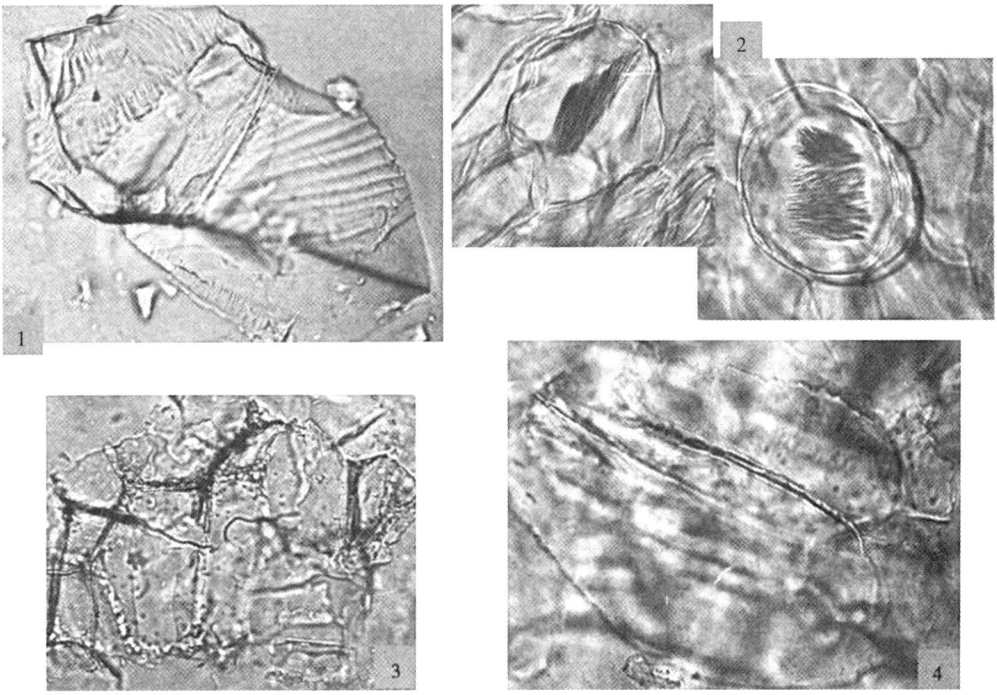

图 32-4　天麻（块茎）粉末

1. 糊化多糖类物　2. 草酸钙针晶　3. 厚壁细胞（表面观）　4. 薄壁细胞

3. 理化鉴别

（1）取本品粉末 1 g，加水 10 ml，浸渍 4 小时，随时振摇，滤过。滤液加碘试液 2～4 滴，显紫红色至酒红色。

（2）醇浸液加米隆试剂（硝酸汞试剂）显玫瑰红色，并有白色絮状沉淀产生。

（3）取粉末 0.2 g，加乙醇 10 ml，加热回流 1 小时，滤过，取滤液 1 ml，置 10 ml 量瓶中，加乙醇稀释至刻度，摇匀，以分光光度法测定，在 270 nm 附近有最大吸收或出现一肩峰；另取滤液 1 ml，置 25 ml 量瓶中，加乙醇稀释至刻度，摇匀，在 219～224 nm 波长范围内有最大吸收。

【实验作业】

1. 绘天麻块茎横切面组织简图。
2. 绘天麻粉末特征图，示厚壁细胞、草酸钙针晶束、多糖团块。
3. 记述天麻理化鉴别的步骤与结果。

【思考题】

1. 天麻的生活史是怎样的？
2. 天麻的主要化学成分是什么？
3. 天麻的伪品有哪些？

32 Identification of Rhizoma Gastrodiae (Orchidaceae)

Objectives

1. Master the description and microscopic identification of Rhizoma Gastrodiae.

2. Master the chemical constituents and physico-chemical identification on Rhizoma Gastrodiae.

3. Study the distinguishing characters of *G. elata* and its adulterants.

Experiment Material

Crude drug specimens of *Gastrodia elata* Bl., permanent mounts of Rhizoma Gastrodiae, powered Rhizoma Gastrodiae

Experiment Methods

1. Description

Ellipsoid or slat-shaped, slightly compressed, shrunken and somewhat curved, 3～15 cm long, 1.5～6 cm wide, 0.5～2 cm thick. Externally yellowish-white to yellowish-brown, with irregular longitudinal wrinkles and many transverse annulations arranged by latent buds, sometimes brown funiculi visible. Apex with reddish-brown to deep brown parrot-beak like buds "Dongma" or remains of stem "Chunma"; the lower end with a rounded scar. Texture hard and uneasily broken, fracture fairly even, yellowish-white to brownish, horny. Odour, slight; taste, sweetish.

2. Microscopic identification

Transverse Section: Remains of epidermis present pale brown. Hypodermis of 2～3 rows of suberized and tangentially elongated cells. Cortex consisting of over 10 rows of polygonal cells, some containing raphides of calcium oxalate. In older tubers 2～3 rows of elliptical sclerenchymatous cells present in cortex adjacent to hypodermis, with lignified and obviously pitted walls. Stele occupied the most part of rhizome, scattered small amphicribral vascular bundles. Parenchymatous cells containing raphides of calcium oxalate.

Powder: Yellowish-white to yellowish brown.

(1) When mounted in Smith's starch reagent, parenchymatous cells containing

gelatinized polysaccharides colourless, and some cells containing long-ovoid, long-ellipsoid or subround granules, showing a brown or brown-purple colour on adding iodine solution.

(2) Needle crystals of calcium oxalate in bundles or scattered, 25～75 (93) μm long.

(3) Sclerenchymatous cells elliptical or subpolygonal, distinctly pitted.

3. Physico-chemical identification

(1) Macerate 1 g of the powder in 10 ml of water for 4 hours with constant shaking and filter. To the filtrate add 2～4 drops of iodine TS, a violet-red to wine-red colour is produced.

(2) Add mercuric nitrate to thanol lixivium, show rose color, and a white flocculent precipitate is produced.

(3) To 0.2 g of the powder add 10 ml of ethanol, heat under reflux for 1 hour, and filter. Transfer 1 ml of filtrate to a 10 ml volumetric flask, dilute with ethanol to volume, and mix well. Carry out the method for spectrophonetry. The light absorption of the solution exhibits a maximum at about 270 nm or a peak with shoulder. Transfer another 1ml of the filtrate to a 25 ml volumetric flask, dilute with ethanol to volume, and mix well. The light absorption of the solution exhibits maximum within the range of 219～224 nm.

Laboratory Assignments

1. Make a drawing of transverse section of Rhizoma Gastrodiae.

2. Make a diagnostic drawing of powder of Rhizome Gastrodiae, and signify the sclerenchymatous cells, raphides of calcium oxalate and amylose conglomeration.

3. Record the procedure and result of physcico-chemical identification on Rhizoma Gastrodiae.

Questions

1. How about the growth cycle of Rhizoma Gastrodiae?

2. What are the major chemical constituents in Rhizoma Gastrodiae?

3. What are the adulterants of Rhizoma Gastrodiae?

实验三十三　兰科生药——石斛的鉴定

【实验目的】

1. 掌握石斛类生药的性状及显微的主要鉴别特征。
2. 熟悉单子叶植物茎的主要鉴别特征。

【实验方法】

金钗石斛 *Dendrobium nobile* Lindl.、环草石斛 *D. loddigesii* Rolfe.、黄草石斛 *D. chrysanthum* Wall.、马鞭石斛 *D. fimbriatum* Hook. var. *oculatum* Hook. 及铁皮石斛 *D. candidum* Wall. ex Lindl. 的生药标本；金钗石斛茎横切片及石斛药材粉末。

【实验方法】

1. 性状鉴别

(1) 金钗石斛：茎下部圆柱形，中上部扁圆柱形，稍曲折略呈“之”字形。节明显，节间长 1.5～6 cm。表面金黄色或绿黄色，有光泽，具深纵沟及纵纹，节膨大，棕色，节上有互生花序柄痕及残存膜质叶鞘。质轻脆，断面较疏松，灰白色，有短纤维状维管束外露。气微，味苦。

(2) 环草石斛：茎细长圆柱形，偶有分枝，常弯曲盘绕成团，节间长 0.5～2.5 cm；金黄色，有光泽，具细纵纹，残留叶鞘松抱于茎，易脱落；质柔韧；味较苦。

(3) 黄草石斛：茎长圆柱形，中上部不规则弯曲，节间长 1～4 cm。表面金黄色至淡黄棕色，具粗细均匀的纵纹，叶鞘有的具紫红色斑点；味微苦，嚼之有黏性。

(4) 铁皮石斛：茎长圆柱形，节间长 1～4 cm，黄色，叶鞘与节间上部留有间隙；经加工成耳环石斛，称“铁皮枫斗”，茎扭曲成螺旋状或弹簧状，一般为 1～5 个旋纹，长 1～5 cm，旋环直径 2～3 mm，一端可见短须根；质坚实，易折断；嚼之有黏性。

(5) 马鞭石斛：茎长圆柱形，节间长 3～4.5 cm。表面黄色至暗黄色，具深纵槽，质疏松，断面纤维性。味微苦。

2. 显微鉴别

(1) 茎横切面

①金钗石斛：扁圆形，边缘有 6～7 个浅波。表皮为 1 列细小扁平细胞，外被厚的角质层。基本薄壁组织中散列多数有限外韧型维管束，略成 7～8 圈；维管束外侧有半月形纤维束，1～4 列，其外缘嵌有细小薄壁细胞，有的含圆簇状硅质块；木质部有 1～4 个导管较大。黏液细胞含草酸钙针晶束，长 50～130 μm。

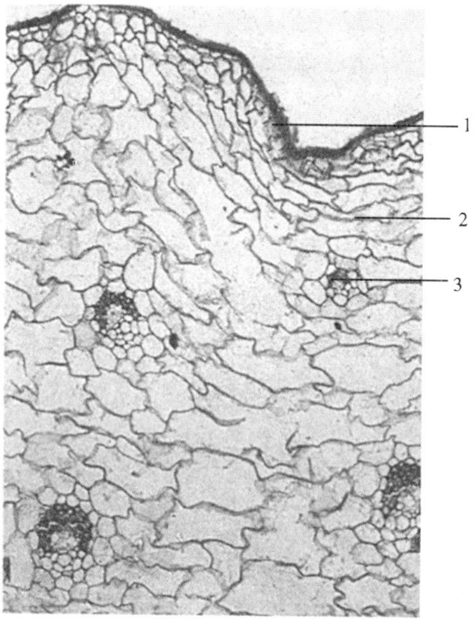

图 33－1　金钗石斛（茎）横切面

1. 表皮　2. 薄壁组织　3. 维管束

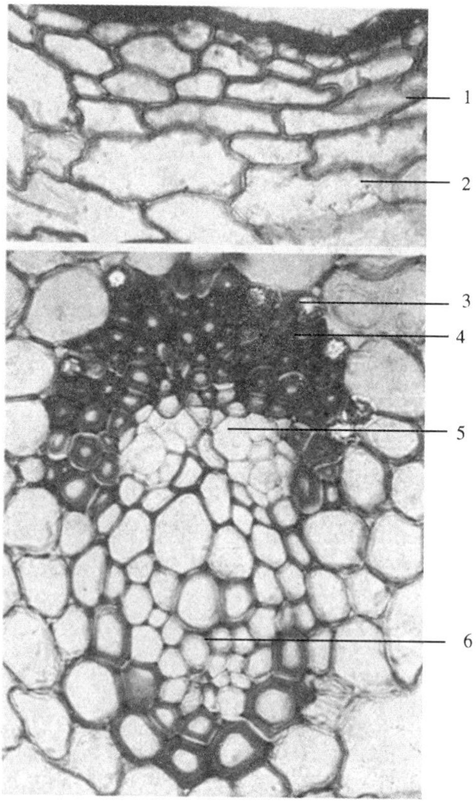

图 33－2　金钗石斛（茎）横切面（局部放大）

1. 表皮　2. 薄壁组织　3. 硅质块　4. 纤维束
5. 韧皮部　6. 木质部

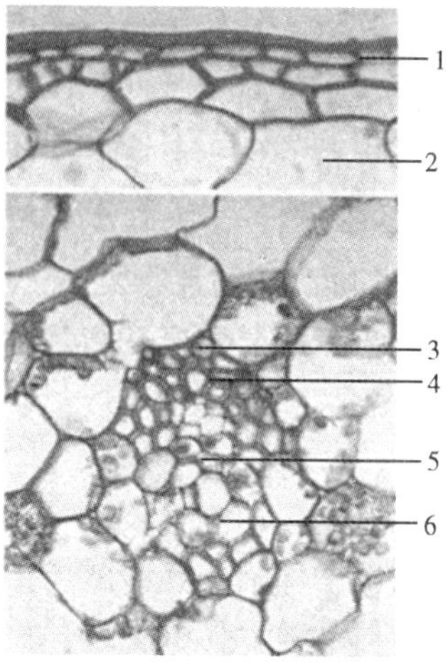

图 33－3　环草石斛（茎）横切面（局部放大）

1. 表皮　2. 薄壁组织　3. 硅质块
4. 纤维束　5. 韧皮部　6. 木质部

②环草石斛：茎横切面维管束略成 3～4 圈；维管束外侧纤维束 2～5 列，含草酸钙针晶细胞多见于维管束旁，针晶束长 50～74 μm。

③黄草石斛：茎横切面维管束略成 5～6 圈；维管束外侧纤维束 1～6 列，硅质块较多，含草酸钙针晶细胞多见于维管束旁，针晶束长 47～83 μm。

④铁皮石斛：维管束略成 4～5 圈；维管束外侧纤维束 1～4 列，含草酸钙针晶细胞多见于近表皮处，针晶束长 60～108 μm。

⑤马鞭石斛：表皮细胞外壁及侧壁增厚，木化，层纹明显，表皮下层厚壁细胞 3～4 列。维管束略成 6～7 圈，维管束外侧纤维束 2～8 列。

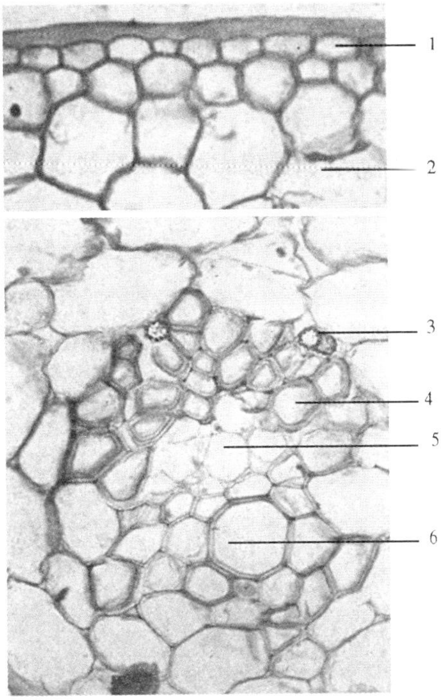

图 33－4　黄草石斛（茎）横切面（局部放大）

1. 表皮　2. 薄壁组织　3. 硅质块　4. 纤维束
5. 韧皮部　6. 木质部

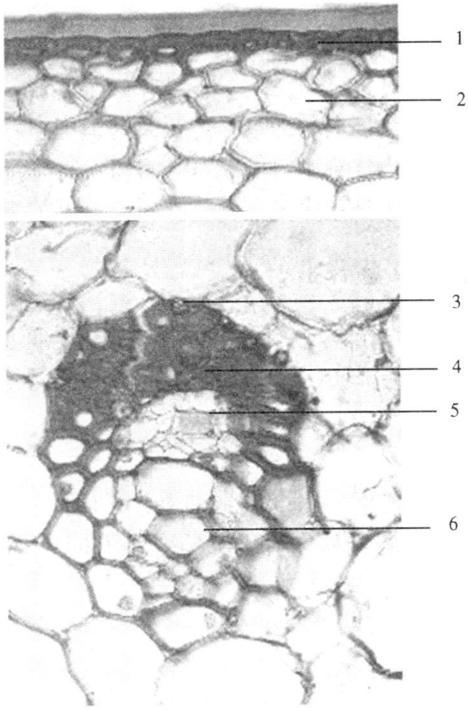

图 33－5　马鞭石斛（茎）横切面（局部放大）

1. 表皮　2. 薄壁组织　3. 硅质块　4. 纤维束
5. 韧皮部　6. 木质部

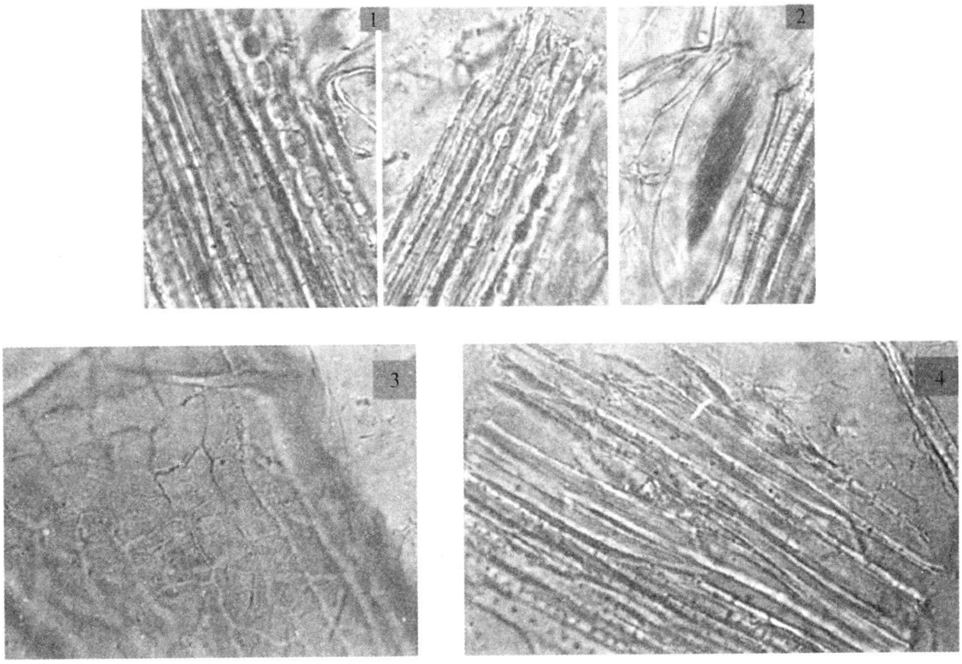

图 33－6　石斛粉末

1. 束鞘纤维　2. 草酸钙针晶　3. 表皮细胞　4. 木纤维

（2）石斛药材粉末：

①束鞘纤维多成束或散离，长梭形，纤维束周围细胞中含类圆形硅质块，含硅质块细胞排成纵行。

②草酸钙针晶束存在于薄壁细胞中，针晶较粗。

③表皮细胞表面观呈长多角形，垂周壁连珠状增厚，角质层表面有网状裂纹。

④木纤维多成束，纹孔较多，可见细小具缘纹孔。

【实验作业】

1. 列表记述石斛类生药的组织特征鉴别要点，并绘金钗石斛茎横切面简图。
2. 绘石斛粉末特征图，示晶鞘纤维、表皮细胞。

【思考题】

1. 如何从性状上区别上述5种石斛？
2. 石斛质量与什么有关？习惯认为枫斗（耳环石斛）为优，为什么？

33 Identification of Caulis Dendrobii (Orchidaceae)

Objectives

1. Master the description and microscopic identification of Caulis Dendrobii.

2. Familiar with the main distinguishing characters of stems from Monocotyledoneae.

Experiment Material

Crude drug specimens of *Dendrobium nobile* Lindl., *D. loddigesii* Rolfe., *D. chrysanthum* Wall, *D. fimbriatum* Hook. var. *oculatum* Hook. and *D. candidum* Wall. ex Lindl.; permanent mounts of stem from *Dendrobium nobile* Lindl. and powder of Caulis Dendrobii.

Experiment Methods

1. Description

(1) Stem of *Dendrobium nobile*: the bottom of stem cylindrical, the middle and top flattened-cylindrical, slightly curved, "Z" -shaped. With distinct nodes, internodes 1.5~6 cm long. Externally golden or greenish-yellow, lustrous, deeply furrowed and striated longitudinally, nodes swollen, brown, bearing stalk scar of alternate inflorescence and membranous leaf sheaths residual. Texture light and fragile, fracture relatively lax, greyish-white, short fibre vascular bundles revealed. Odour slight, taste bitter.

(2) Stem of *D. loddigesii*: stem slenderly cylindrical, occasionally branched, frequently curved and rolled into masses, internodes 0.5 ~ 2.5 cm long; golden, lustrous, finely striated longitudinally, leaf sheaths residual amplexicaul laxly, easily dropped; texture pliable and solid; taste relatively bitter.

(3) Stem of *D. chrysanthum*: stem long-cylindrical, the middle-top irregularly curved, internodes 1~4 cm long. Externally golden to pale yellowish-brown, furrowed longitudinally and even, leaf sheaths sometimes with purplish-red spots; taste slightly bitter, viscous on chewing.

(4) Stem of *D. candidum*: stem long-cylindrical, internodes 1~4 cm, yellow, flaws between leaf sheaths and the top of internodes; processed to Erhuanshihu, named

" Tiepi Fengdow". Stem twisted to spiral or spring-like, usually with 1~5 spires, 1~5 cm long, 2~3 mm in diameter, at one end some short fibrous roots remained; texture compact, easily broken; viscous on chewing.

(5) Stem of *D. fimbriatum* var. *oculatum*: stem long-cylindrical, internodes 3~4.5 cm long. Externally yellow to dark yellow, deeply grooved longitudinally, texture laxly, fracture fibrous, taste slightly bitter.

2. Microscopic identification

(1) Transverse section of stem

Dendrobium nobile: flattened-rounded, 6~7 shallow waves on the edge. Epidermal cells of 1 layer small and flattened, covered with thick cuticle. Basic parenchymatous tissues, scattered with numerous closed collateral vascular bundles, somewhat arranged in 7 ~ 8 whorls; fibre bundles at the outer side of vascular bundles crescent or semicircular, 1~4 layers, small parenchymatous cells at the outer side part containing subround silica bodies; xylem with 1~4 relatively large vessels. Mucus cells containing needle crystal bundles of calcium oxalate, 50~130 μm long.

D. loddigesii: vascular bundles somewhat arranged in 3~4 whorls; fibre bundles at the outer side of vascular bundles 2~5 layers, most of cells containing needle crystals of calcium oxalate accompanied by vascular bundles, needle crystal bundles 50~74 μm long.

D. chrysanthum: vascular bundles somewhat arranged in 5 ~ 6 whorls; fibre bundles at the outer side of vascular bundles 1 ~ 6 layers, more silica bodies, most of cells containing needle crystals of calcium oxalate accompanied by vascular bundles, needle crystal bundles 47~83 μm long.

D. candidum: vascular bundles somewhat arranged in 4~5 whorls; fibre bundles at the outer side of vascular bundles 1 ~ 4 layers, most of cells containing needle crystals of calcium oxalate occurring near the epidermis, needle crystal bundles 60~108 μm long.

D. fimbriatum var. *oculatum*: epidermal cells outer walls and lateral walls thickened, lignified and distinctly striated, underneath epidermis 3 ~ 4 layers of thickwalled-cells. Vascular bundles somewhat arranged in 6~7 whorls, fibre bundles at the outer side of vascular bundles 2~8 layers.

(2) Powder of Caulis Dendrobii

① Fibres out side of vascular bundles mostly in bundles or scattered, long-shuttled, cells around fiber bundles containing subrounded silica bodies, arranged in rows longitudinally.

② Needle crystal bundles of calcium oxalate occurring in parenchymatous cells, needle crystals relatively thick.

③ Epidermal cells in surface view long-polygon, anticlinal walls beaded thickened, chicken wire cracking on the surface of cuticle.

④ Woody fibre mostly in bundles, pits more, with small bordered pits.

Laboratory Assignments

1. Make a table to record distinguishing points of Genus *Dendrobium*, and draw a drawing of transverse section of stem from *Dendrobium nobile*.

2. Draw characteristic drawings of the powder of Caulis Dendrobii, and signify the crystal fibres, epidermal cells.

Questions

1. How to distinct the mentioned five kinds of crude drugs from Genus *Dendrobium* by description?

2. What are related to the quality of Caulis Dendrobii? Why is it used to believe that Fengdou (Erhuanshihu) was the best?

实验三十四　动物类生药——斑蝥的鉴定

【实验目的】

1. 掌握斑蝥的性状鉴别特征。
2. 掌握斑蝥的化学成分及理化鉴别方法。

【实验材料】

南方大斑蝥 *Mylabris phalerata* Pallas 或黄黑小斑蝥 *M. cichorii* L. 的生药标本及斑蝥粉末。

【实验方法】

1. 性状鉴别

南方大斑蝥：虫体呈长圆形，长 1.5～2.5 cm，宽 0.5～1 cm，头及口器下垂，有较大的复眼及触角各 1 对，触角多已脱落。背部具革质鞘翅 1 对，黑色，有黄色或棕黄色横纹 3 条，鞘翅下有棕色膜状透明的内翅 2 片。胸腹部乌黑色，有光泽，胸部有足 3 对。有特殊异臭。

黄黑小斑蝥：体型较小，长 1～1.5 cm。

1　　2　　3

图 34－1　斑蝥薄层层析图谱

1. 斑蝥素　2. 斑蝥（对照药材）　3. 斑蝥（商品）

2. 理化鉴别

（1）粉末进行微量升华，得柱形或棱形斑蝥素结晶。

①将升华物用石油醚洗 2～3 次，加硫酸 2～3 滴，微热溶解，转入试管内，小火加热至发生气泡，稍冷，加二甲氨基苯甲醛硫酸溶液 1 滴，显樱红色或紫红色。

②将升华物加硫酸 2～3 滴，微热溶解，转入试管内，加间苯二酚粉末少许，小火加热至沸，溶液显红色，在紫外灯下观察显绿色荧光。

③将升华物滴加氢氧化钡水溶液封藏后镜检，可见斑蝥酸钡盐的针晶束。

（2）薄层层析　取斑蝥粉末 3 g，加三氯甲烷 20 ml，振摇，浸泡 2 小时，过滤，滤液蒸干，残渣用石油醚（30～60℃）洗 3 次，每次 5 ml，小心倾去上清液，残渣加三氯甲烷 1 ml 使溶解，作供试品溶液。另取斑蝥素对照品，加三氯甲烷制成每 1ml 含 5mg 的溶液，作对照品溶液。吸取上述两种溶液各 5 μl，分别点于同一硅胶 G 薄层板，以三氯甲烷:丙酮（49:1）为展开剂，展开，取出，晾干，喷0.1%溴甲酚绿乙醇试液，110℃加热至斑点显色清晰。供试品色谱中，在与对照品色谱相应位置上显1个黄色斑点。

【实验作业】

记述理化鉴别实验的操作步骤及结果。

【思考题】

1. 如何鉴别斑蝥和青娘子，两者在功效上有何不同？
2. 根据斑蝥素的化学结构，如何改造使其毒性降低？

34 Identification of Mylabris

Objectives

1. Master the description of Mylabris.

2. Master the chemical constituents and physico-chemical identification on Mylabris.

Experiment Material

Crude drug specimens of *Mylabris phalerata* Pallas or *M. cichorii* Linnaeus and powder of Mylabris.

Experiment Methods

1. Description

Mylabris phalerata: body elongated round, 1.5～2.5 cm long, 0.5～1 cm wide, the head and the mouth parts curved downward, with a pair of relatively large compound eyes and a pair of antennae which usually fallen off. A pair of leathery elytra on the dorsum, black, with three yellow or brownish-yellow transverse stripes, a pair of transparent brownish membrane-like hind wings beneath the elytra. The thorax and abdomen pitch-black, with three pairs of legs at the thorax. Odour characteristic stinking.

Mylabris cichorii: body size relatively small, 1～1.5 cm long.

2. Physico-chemical identification

(1) Columnar or arris crystals of cantharidin from the microsublimation of the powder.

①Wash the sublimate 2～3 times with petroleum ether, add 2～3 drops of sulfuric acid, heat and dissolve, then transfer to a tube, heat gently to effervesce, cool, add 1 drop of dimethylaminobenzaldehyde sulfuric acid solution, a cherryish-red or purplish-red colour is produced.

②To the sublimate add 2～3 drops of sulfuric acid, heat, dissolve and transfer to a tube, add a small quantity of resorcinol powder, heat gently to boil, a red colour is produced, under viltalight lamp with green fluoranthene.

③Mount the sublimate in barium hydroxide and examine, needle crystal bundles of barium salt of cantharis acid can be observed.

(2) TLC: To 3 g of the powder add 20 ml of chloroform, shake, macerate for 2 hours, and filter, evaporate the filtrate to dryness, wash the residue with 3 quantities, each of 5 ml of petroleum ether (30～60℃), carefully discard the supernatant, dissolve the residue in 1 ml of chloroform as the test solution. Dissolve cantharidin CRS in chloroform to produce a solution containing 5 mg per ml as the reference solution. Using silica gel G as the coating substance and chloroform-acetone (49 : 1) as the mobile phase. Apply separately 5 μl of each of the two solutions to the plate. After developing and removal of the plate, dry it in air. Spray with a 0.1% solution of bromocresol virid in ethanol and heat in 110℃ to the spots distinct. The spot is yellow, the spot in the chromatogram obtained with the test solution corresponds in position and colour to the spot in the chromatogram obtained with the reference solution.

Laboratory Assignments

Record the procedure and result of physico-chemical experiments.

Questions

1. How to identify Mylabris and Lytta? What are the differences between the two in action?

2. According to the chemical structure of cantharidin, how to reform it to diminish toxicity?

实验三十五　动物类生药——僵蚕的鉴定

【实验目的】

1. 掌握僵蚕性状、显微的主要鉴别特征。
2. 了解动物类生药的鉴别特征。

【实验材料】

僵蚕［家蚕 *Bombyx mori* L.4～5 龄的幼虫因感染白僵菌 *Beauveria bassiana*（Bals.）Vuillant 而致死的干燥虫体］的生药标本及僵蚕粉末。

【实验内容】

1. 性状鉴别

虫体类圆柱形，多弯曲皱缩，长 2～5 cm，直径 5～7 mm。表面灰白色或黄白色，被有白色粉霜状的气生菌丝及分生孢子；头部较圆，黄棕色；体节明显，尾部略呈二歧状；短足 8 对，略呈突起状。质硬脆，断面平坦，外层白色，显粉性，中间有亮棕色或亮黑色的丝腺环 4 个。气微腥，味微咸。

2. 显微鉴别

僵蚕粉末：

（1）菌丝近无色，细长弯曲，相互盘缠交织附于体壁。

（2）气管壁碎片具棕色或深棕色螺旋丝。

（3）表皮表面有极皱缩的网络样纹理及纹理突起形成的小尖突，尖突较密集；毛窝类圆形，边缘黄棕色；刚毛黄色或黄棕色，表面光滑，壁厚。

（4）未消化桑叶组织，可见含钟乳体表皮细胞或短腺毛；叶肉细胞含草酸钙簇晶、方晶及细小杆状结晶。

【实验作业】

简述僵蚕性状与显微鉴别特征，并绘显微特征图，示菌丝、气管碎片、表皮表面观。

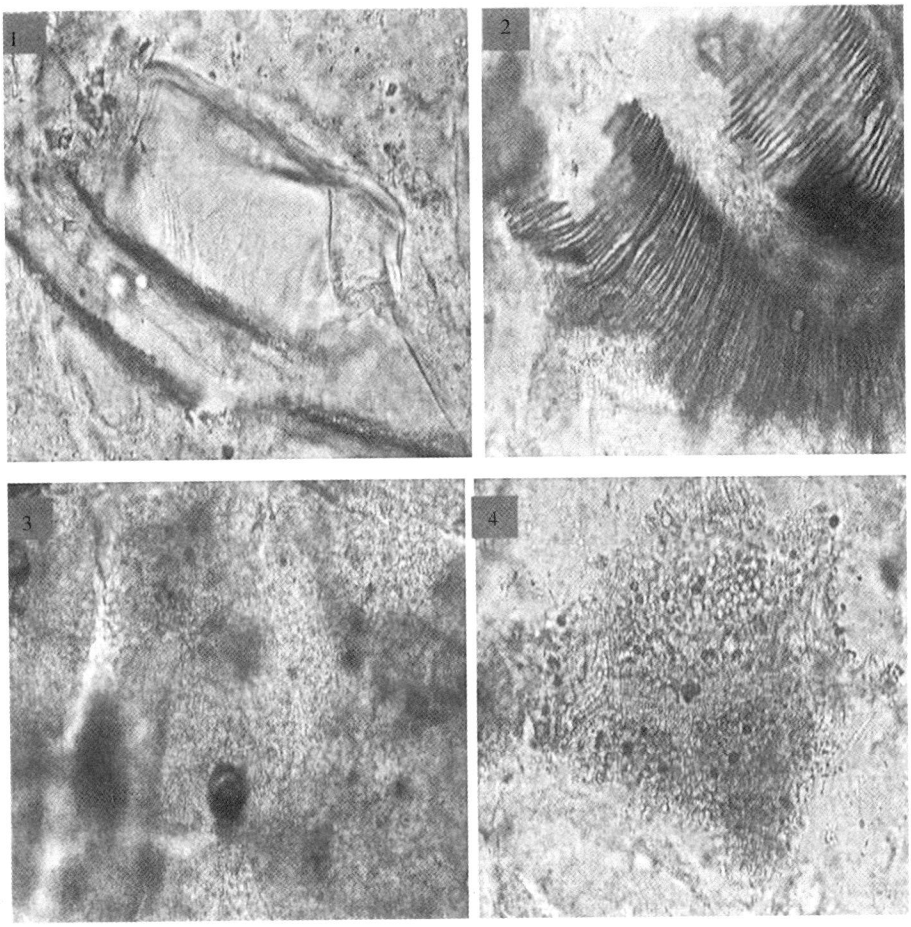

图 35-1　僵蚕粉末

1. 菌丝　2. 气管碎片　3. 表皮　4. 未消化桑叶组织

35 Identification of Bombyx Batryticatus

Objectives

1. Master the description and microscopic identification of Bombyx Batryticatus.
2. Study the distinguishing characters of animal drugs.

Experiment Material

Crude drug specimens of Bombyx Batryticatus [the dried body of the 4 ~ 5 stage larva of *Bombyx mori* L. died of infection (or artificial infection) of *Beauveria bassiana* (Bals.) Vuillant] and powder of Bombyx Batryticatus.

Experiment Methods

1. Description

Somewhat cylindric, usually curved and shrunken, 2 ~ 5 cm long, 5 ~ 7 mm in diameter. The surface grayish-white or yellowish-white, covered with white powdery aerial mycelia and conidia; the head relatively round, yellowish-brown; body nodes conspicuous, caudal portion somewhat dichotomic; 8 pairs of short legs, segments prominent. Texture hard and fragile, fracture even, peripheral layer white, powdery, middle part with 4 bright brown or bright black rings of silk glands. Odour slightly stinking, taste slightly salty.

2. Microscopic identification

Powder of Bombyx Batryticatus:

(1) The mycelia almost colourless, slender rolled and twisted in the body walls.

(2) Broken pieces of the trachea walls with brown or dark brown spiral filaments.

(3) The surface of the epidermis with reticulated shrunken striations and small pointed projections formed by the striations, relatively dense; with rounded setae pits, the margin of the pits yellowish-brown; setae yellow or yellowish-brown, surface smooth, walls thickened.

(4) The indigested mulberry leaf tissues, containing epidermal cells with cistolith or short glandular hairs; leaf flesh cells containing clusters, prisms or small rod-shaped

crytals of calcium oxalate.

Laboratory Assignments

Describe briefly the description and microscopic identification of Bombyx Batryticatus, draw the drawing of microscopic characteristic, and signify the mycelia, broken pieces of the trachea and epidermis in surface view.

实验三十六 矿物类生药——朱砂、石膏的鉴定

【实验目的】

1. 掌握朱砂及石膏的性状及理化鉴别方法。
2. 熟悉矿物类生药的性状鉴别方法。

【实验材料】

朱砂 Cinnabaris；石膏 Gypsum Fibrosum。

【实验方法】

1. 朱砂的鉴别

(1) 性状鉴别

朱砂为粒状或块状集合体，呈颗粒状或块片状。鲜红色或暗红色，条痕朱红色至红褐色，具光泽。体重，质脆，片状者易破碎，粉末状者有闪烁的光泽，气微，无味。

(2) 理化鉴别

①取朱砂粉末，用盐酸湿润后，在光洁的铜片上摩擦，铜片表面显银白色光泽，加热烘烤后，银白色即消失。

②取朱砂粉末 2 g，加盐酸－硝酸（3∶1）的混合溶液 2 ml 使溶解，蒸干，加水 2 ml 使溶解，滤过，收集滤液。

取滤液，加氢氧化钠试液，即生成黄色沉淀。

取滤液，加碘化钾试液，即生成猩红色沉淀，加过量的碘化钾试液，沉淀溶解，用氢氧化钠碱化后再加氯化铵试液即生成红棕色沉淀。

取滤液，加氯化钡试液，即生成白色沉淀。分离出沉淀，加盐酸，沉淀不溶解。

取滤液，加醋酸铅试液，即生成白色沉淀。分离沉淀，加醋酸铵试液，沉淀溶解。

2. 石膏的鉴别

(1) 性状鉴别

石膏为纤维状的集合体，呈长块状、板块状或不规则块状。白色、灰白色或淡黄色，有的半透明。体重，质软，纵断面具绢丝样光泽。气微，味淡。

(2) 理化鉴别

①取本品一小块（约 2 g），置具有小孔软木塞的试管内，灼烧，管壁有水生成，小块变为不透明体。

②用铂丝，以盐酸润湿后，蘸取石膏粉末，在无色火焰中燃烧，火焰即显砖红色。

③取本品粉末 0.2 g，加稀盐酸 10 ml，加热使溶解，加甲基红指示液 2 滴，用氨试液中和，再滴加盐酸至恰呈酸性，加草酸铵试液，即生成白色沉淀；分离沉淀，加醋酸，沉淀不溶解；加盐酸沉淀溶解。

【实验作业】

1. 描述所观察的朱砂、石膏性状特征。
2. 记录朱砂、石膏的理化鉴别过程与结果。

【思考题】

1. 什么是矿物类生药的本色、外色、假色、条痕色?
2. 矿物类生药的硬度是如何确定的?

36 Identification of Cinnabaris and Gypsum Fibrosum

Objectives

1. Master the description and physico-chemical identification on Cinnabaris and Gypsum Fibrosum.

2. Familiar with the description of mineral drugs.

Experiment Material

Cinnabaris, Gypsum Fibrosum.

Experiment Methods

1. Identification of Cinnabaris

(1) Description

Aggregates of granulous or lumpy masses, in granules or pieces. Bright red or dark red, streak red to brownish-red, lustrous. Texture heavy and fragile, pieces easily broken and granules with glittering gloss. Odourless and tasteless.

(2) Physico-chemical Identification

① Moisten the powder with hydrochloric acid, rub on a clean surface of copper slice, the surface shows the silver gloss, which disappear immediately on heating.

② Dissolve 2 g of Cinnabris powder in 2 ml of a mixture of hydrochloric acid-nitric acid (3 : 1), evaporate to dryness, dissolve the residue in 2 ml of water and filter, collect the filtrate.

To the filtrate add sodium hydroxide solution, yellow precipitate is produced.

To the filtrate add potassium iodide solution, scarlet red precipitate is produced, which is soluble in an excess of reagent, add sodium hydroxide to basic capacity, then reddish-brown precipitate is produced on addition of ammonium chloride.

To the filtrate add barium chloride, white precipitate is produced, which is insoluble on addition of hydrochloric acid.

To the filtrate add lead acetate solution, white precipitate is produced, which dissolves on addition of ammonium acetate solution.

2. Identification of Gypsum Fibrosum

(1) Description

Fibrous aggregates in long, plate-shaped or irregular pieces, white, greyish-white or pale yellow, sometimes translucent. Texture heavy and soft, longitudinally cut surface with silky luster. Odourless; taste weak.

(2) Physico-chemical Identification

① Ignite a piece of the drug (about 2 g) in a test tube covered with a pored cork stopper, the moisture is produced on the tube wall and the small piece turns to opaque.

② Moisten the substance being examined with hydrochloric acid on a platinum wire, it imparts a yellowish-red colour to a nonluminous flame

③ To 0.2 g of the powder add 10 ml of dilute hydrochloric acid, heat to dissolve, add 2 drops of methyl red indicator, neutralize with ammonium solution, then acidify with hydrochloric acid. Add ammonium oxalate TS, a white precipitate is produced, which is insoluble in acetate acid but soluble in hydrochloric acid.

Laboratory Assignments

1. Describe the description of Cinnabaris and Gypsum Fibrosum examined.

2. Record the procedure and result of physico-chemical identification of Cinnabaris and Gypsum Fibrosum.

Questions

1. What are the intricate colour, exo-colour, false colour and streak colour of mineral drugs?

2. How to determine hardness number of mineral drugs?